MenuPause

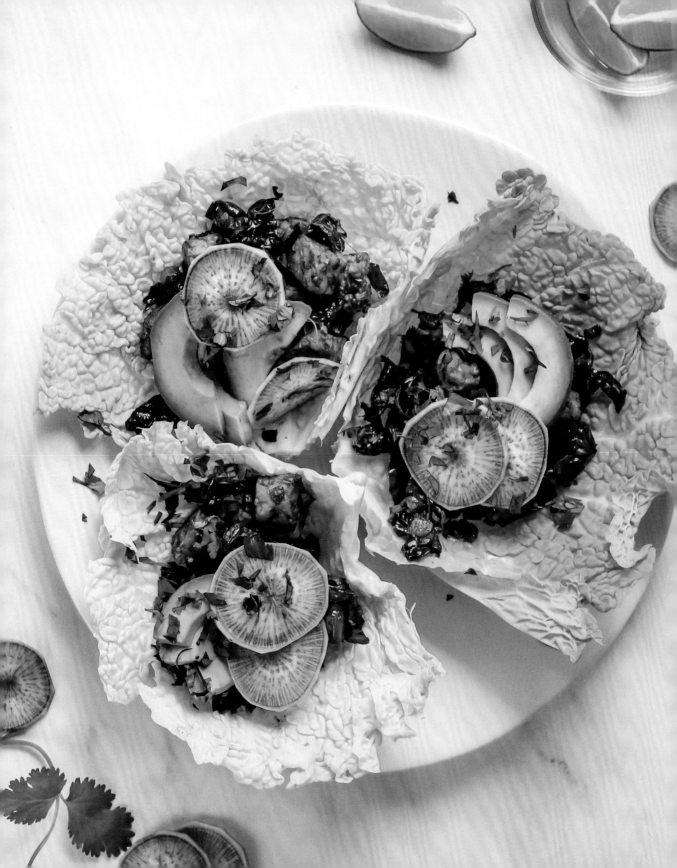

MenuPause

Five Unique Eating Plans to Break Through Your Weight Loss
Plateau and Improve Mood, Sleep, and Hot Flashes

Anna Cabeca, DO, OBGYN, FACOG

RODALE.

NEW YORK

Also by Dr. Anna Cabeca

The Hormone Fix

Keto-Green 16

Published in the United States by Rodale Books, an imprint of Random House, a division of Penguin Random House LLC, New York.
rodalebooks.com

RODALE and the Plant colophon are registered trademarks of Penguin Random House LLC.

Library of Congress Cataloging-in-Publication Data
Names: Cabeca, Anna, author.
Title: Menupause : five unique eating plans to break through your weight loss plateau and improve mood, sleep, and hot flashes / Anna Cabeca, DO, OBGYN, FACOG.
Description: New York : Rodale, [2022] | Includes bibliographical references and index.
Identifiers: LCCN 2021016766 (print) | LCCN 2021016767 (ebook) | ISBN 9780593234495 (hardcover) | ISBN 9780593234501 (ebook)
Subjects: LCSH: Menopause--Diet therapy--Popular works. | Menopause--Nutritional aspects--Popular works. | Menopause--Complications--Diet therapy--Recipes.
Classification: LCC RG186 .C223 2022 (print) | LCC RG186 (ebook) | DDC 618.1/750654--dc23

ISBN 978-0-593-23449-5
Ebook ISBN 978-0-593-23450-1

Printed in China

Editor: Marnie Cochran
Designer: Jennifer K. Beal Davis
Production Editor: Serena Wang
Production Manager: Kim Tyner
Composition: Merri Ann Morrell, Nick Patton, and Zoe Tokushige
Copy Editor: Carole Berglie
Indexer: Jay Kreider

10 9 8 7 6 5 4 3 2 1

First Edition

It is in the pauses of our lives that we find the magic!

To my daughters Brittany, Amanda, Amira,
and Avamarie, and to my son Garrett in heaven—
my days start with gratitude for you.

To my cousin Grace and all women like you
who have struggled to find the next right step for
optimal health. This book is for you.

To all the women in my Girlfriend Doctor Club,
for sharing your stories and journeys and building
a loving community. I am full of gratitude for all of you.

Contents

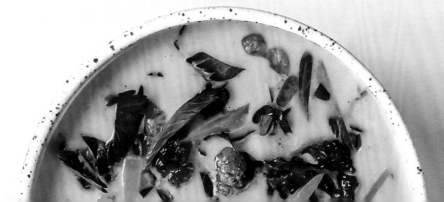

PART 3—THE *MENUPAUSE* RECIPES

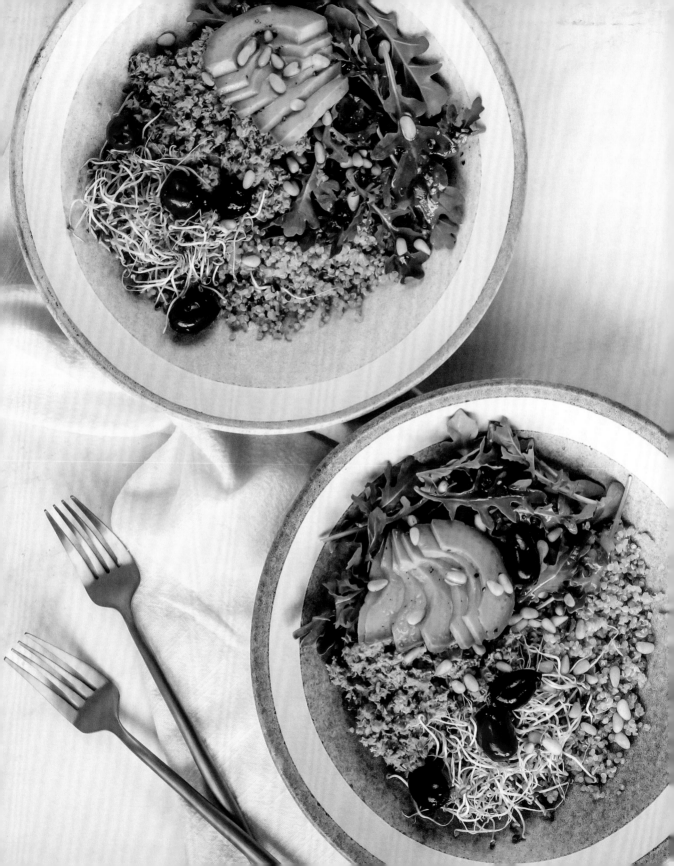

Introduction

Welcome to the process of reclaiming your health and your life through food that both tastes great and is great for your body. In so doing, you are joining a family of like-minded women—women who have "gathered" on my Facebook communities and who take part in the Girlfriend Doctor Club via my website. Our shared goal is to support one another openly and honestly through various life stages, including—and mostly—menopause, which can be the most challenging time of your life.

Let's be honest, ladies: the hormonal fluctuation that precipitates menopause wreaks havoc on our otherwise normal and happy lives. I know, and I can relate. I've been through it not once but twice. The first time I was 39. My toddler son was killed in a tragic accident and the ensuing stress, lack of sleep, and bone-deep sadness effectively stopped my periods. It plunged me into what doctors diagnosed as an "early menopause." Menopause wasn't even on my mind—I was certain it happened mostly to women who were 50-plus years old. Then came the symptoms, starting with weight gain. I had struggled with my weight all my life, once being well over 240 pounds. This was all so frightening, and I wasn't ready, nor did I feel capable of dealing with it.

Eventually (no thanks to anything that any doctor did for me!), I was able to reverse my early menopause and, miraculously, I had another baby. But then I got to 48 years old, closer to the start of the traditional menopause age range, and it all began to happen again, only worse. This time, my joints ached, I slept less and struggled with depression, and I had a hard time zipping up most of my clothes. I felt betrayed by my body. The experience was like PMS on steroids, and I couldn't be sure when *or if* it would ever end.

Both times, it took all my willpower to get my hormones and life in order. I remember hitting such a low point that I didn't want to get out of bed. But I needed progress. I needed to feel better, I had to.

And I did.

The way I did it was through natural means—primarily nutrition and lifestyle! Yes, my entire approach to self-care started with food. I cut out all gluten, refined sugars, and processed foods, and I upped my protein, green veggies, and healthy fats. I refined my supplement intake. I began journaling how I felt, which helped me confirm that food was healing me in truly great ways.

Soon, I began to feel terrific, whole again, and ready to engage life, full steam ahead. I went on to create online programs

Opposite: Salmon Quinoa Bowl, page 263

to help women balance their hormones and heal their bodies. I wrote two books on the issue—*The Hormone Fix* and *Keto-Green 16*—which featured plans to help women (men, too) overcome the almost-universal fallout from hormonal changes: weight gain. And I've developed platforms like my website (dranna.com), podcasts, and *The Girlfriend Doctor Show* to spread healing and support to women everywhere.

My diets and these programs have succeeded beyond my expectations. They are responsible for tens of thousands of women preventing and reversing menopause symptoms, along with losing weight safely and easily—all while rebalancing their hormones.

Which brings me to *MenuPause*. This is a novel cookbook filled with tasty, satisfying recipes, along with five breakthrough 6-day diet plans backed by self-care guidelines to help you on your healing journey. The variety of plans are to help you break free of a plateau and accelerate results. Just like you have to change your exercise routine, you have to change your eating routine. My goal in writing this cookbook is to share with you how delicious, nutritious foods will ease your symptoms and help you achieve amazing well-being. This cookbook will help you discover the quality and variety of flavorful dishes so that you can live a fulfilling life, a life in which you wake up every day, loving the woman you have become.

All health begins with nutrient-rich foods. This is not a new concept, of course. Since ancient times, food has been central to medicine and healing, as well as to illness prevention. The father of medicine, Hippocrates, is to thank for the famous quote: "Let food be thy medicine and medicine be thy food." Food was the first medicine used in ancient times to restore harmony in someone who was ill. And it still works wonders today.

Women in other parts of the world know this! Many of us in the Western world approach menopause with fear and dread: weight gain, insomnia, brain fog, anxiety, depression, hot flashes, loss of libido, loss of memory, and more. Not coincidentally, we suffer greater menopausal symptoms than other women around the globe. Is our diet to blame? Very much so!

After my precious son died, my family and I took a trip around the world. One of my missions was to discover the very best natural practices of healers all over the globe—practices I could incorporate into my life and into the lives of women everywhere. On this worldwide journey, I discovered that menopause and other phases of women's lives cause fewer symptoms elsewhere than they do in American women. An older woman is revered, listened to, and respected for her wisdom.

Why is this? Because menopause in other cultures is treated with natural methods— with diet being the number-one way to reduce symptoms and ease the transition.

Yes, diet! Dietary steps and other lifestyle changes not only make menopause more manageable but also perimenopause and postmenopause.

So, as added features in this cookbook, I include sections called "Menopause Around the World," illustrating how women in other countries go through natural menopause and have very few menopause-related complications. It is believed that their natural, hormone-balancing diets, as well as high levels of physical activity, help reduce the negative effects of menopause. And many women in these cultures have naturally high levels of sex hormones, like estrogen, DHEA (dehydroepiandrosterone), and progesterone as they age—levels that are higher than those of American women of the same age. Again, the reason has to do with diet, but also with maintaining a positive outlook. Although women in other countries experience stress, they've created cultures to cope with it, including having supportive communities, multi-generational households, and a deep sense of spirituality, meaning, and purpose. This is certainly true in the Blue Zones—areas of the world with the highest numbers of people over 100 years old.

There's nothing to say that we can't develop the same powerful lifestyles and attitudes. Toward that end, I've created many recipes that reflect cultures in which the transition to menopause is largely symptom free and a time to be celebrated.

When you learn how to prepare yummy meals filled with healing nutrients—rather than relying on convenience or processed foods—you take giant leaps forward to feeling and looking your best, and that's for a lifetime. When you know how to cook healthful meals, you will heal your menopausal symptoms. When you start enjoying this way of living, you walk into a

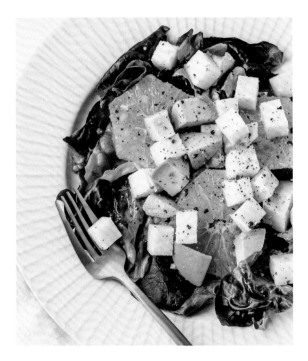

life full of happiness and wholeness—a life you deserve.

MenuPause is about upending the way you eat, cementing new food habits, and taking care of your health and excess weight. It is all about eating real foods. Fresh, organic foods. Foods that are full of nutrients, good proteins, and healing fats that keep your body in peak health. Frankly, this food is good for you no matter what your age or stage in life. And your whole family can enjoy it with you!

But for women in the throes of peri-menopause or menopause, I've seen near-miraculous changes. They were feeling ill, fatigued, and out of sorts, suffering from depression and anxiety, and burdened with excess pounds. But once they changed their nutrition, they

Above: Jicama Salad, page 177

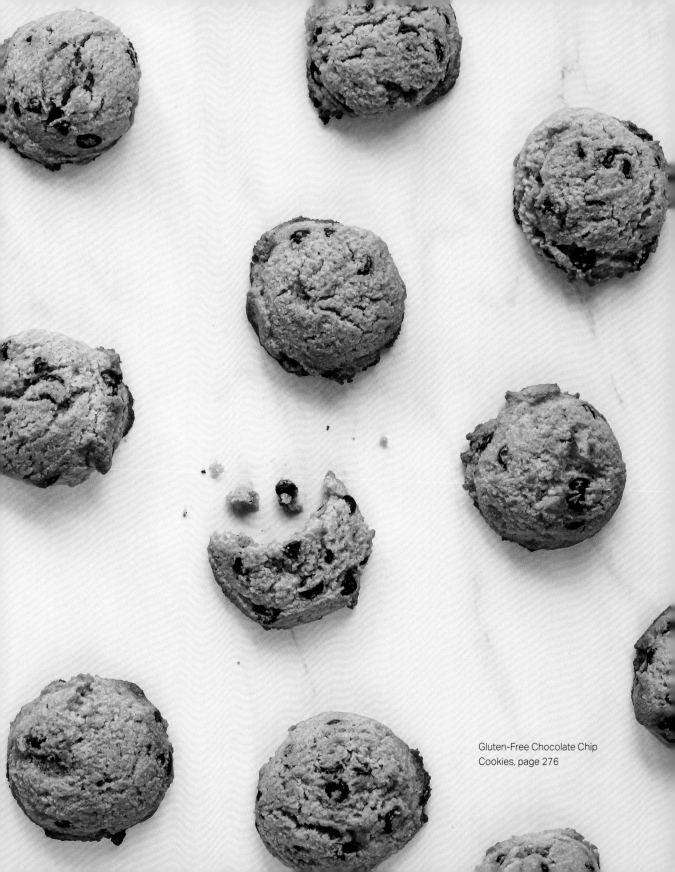

Gluten-Free Chocolate Chip
Cookies, page 276

got sexy and slim, their moods brightened, their thoughts sharpened, their bodies strengthened—and more.

These are all the benefits of the kind of eating you'll learn about in these pages. The doable 6-day plans and accompanying recipes will help you with the following:

- Take off pounds quickly, drop a dress size in under a week, or get in shape for an event coming up that you want to look your best for, or stay at your dream weight if you're already there.

- Understand how weight gain affects and worsens the most common symptoms of menopause: hot flashes, night sweats, insomnia, irritability, anxiety, depression, fatigue, and brain fog. If you're struggling with being overweight, your other symptoms will be even rougher. But if you can get your weight under control, your journey through menopause will be a smooth one. For this reason, I devote a lot of time in this cookbook to the relationship between weight and menopause.

- Overcome a frustrating condition called "weight-loss resistance," in which you can't seem to drop even a pound or your weight comes off too slowly.

- Tackle and overcome unsettling symptoms like hot flashes, night sweats, poor sleep, depression, and irritability.

- Reset your body if you've been overindulging too long in the wrong foods, or suffering burnout from an overly hectic lifestyle, both physically and mentally.

- Rebalance your hormones, whether you're in perimenopause, menopause, or postmenopause.

- Detox yourself from alcohol, caffeine, processed foods, and animal foods that are full of antibiotics and hormones.

- Pause from certain foods and substances that are keeping you unwell.

- Help resolve chronic illnesses such as autoimmune diseases, inflammation, pain, and other issues related to menopause and aging.

- Help prevent menopause-related conditions such as heart disease, diabetes, osteoporosis, even certain cancers.

Whatever your age, whatever your needs, this cookbook is for you. I hope you will also use it as a resource for flexible meal planning centered on your specific needs: weight loss, hormone healing, detoxification, and more.

I love the *MenuPause* way of eating. Its "pauses" give us time to reflect, heal, introspect, and cherish what is truly important in our lives. They also break plateaus and keep us on track on our menopausal healing journey. They work wonders and make us feel revitalized physically, mentally, and emotionally. *MenuPause* is where the magic begins.

Welcome to the family with much love!

—Dr. Anna Cabeca,
The Girlfriend Doctor

PART I

The Magic Begins

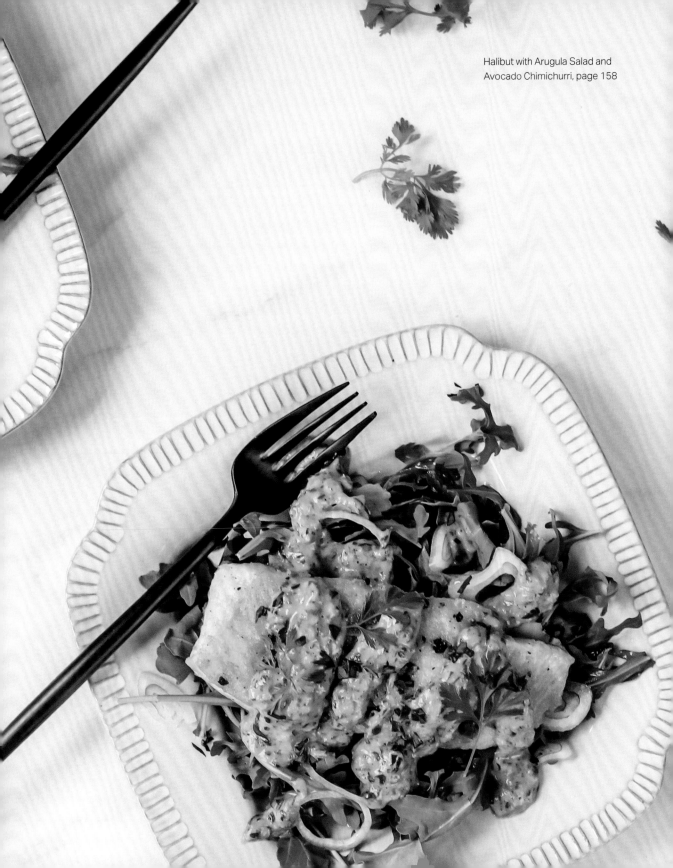

Halibut with Arugula Salad and
Avocado Chimichurri, page 158

CHAPTER 1

Pause a Few Things on Your Menu to End Your Menopausal Symptoms

It is in the pauses of our lives that we find the magic!

Perhaps you picked up this book because you're starting to notice—or long ago noticed!—that your body is changing. Maybe you've gained weight, are having trouble sleeping at night, or are feeling foggy, cranky, and lethargic during the day. What's going on?

If you're nearing the average age of menopause, usually around age 51, or even 10 years earlier, or past the age of 35, there's a simple explanation for these changes: your hormone production has begun to decline. But I know that this medical explanation doesn't help much in the heat of the moment.

Speaking of heat, yes, many of us get those hot flashes and flushes in spades. You feel like you're about to spontaneously burst into a ball of flames at any given moment. Your private lady parts become as dry as the Sahara Desert. You're scared that you've closed up shop as a sexual being.

The seesaw that is your mood has you laughing one instant, sobbing the next, and in the end you just want to sit in the corner with a huge bowl of chocolate ice cream topped with chocolate fudge, chocolate sprinkles, and chocolate-covered nuts. Let me be real here: chocolate *is* generally good for you, but maybe not in such profuse amounts. And the creeping pounds? Oh, my, how we hate muffin tops, and just the fact that we're spreading in weird places, like our tummies and our backs. In fact, we can be doing everything right, which has kept us healthy for years, and yet it has all stopped working.

Beyond these unpleasant symptoms, there's the scary long-term stuff to worry about: once you've reached menopause, you're at higher risk for heart disease, diabetes, certain cancers, osteoporosis, and autoimmune disease.

Now here's the good news—no, the really good news: as expected and as natural as hormonal decline is, there are easy actions you can take to help relieve and prevent these deficiencies, create a higher quality of life, stop negative health outcomes, and

Creamy Coconut-Saffron
Mussels, page 217

reverse other age-related changes. These actions involve *pausing* certain substances that damage our health and worsen symptoms as we go through various life stages. I always tell patients that although menopause is natural, suffering is optional. This is what *MenuPause* is all about.

Examples of substances to pause include the following:

- Carbohydrates
- Excess calories
- Added sugar
- Processed foods
- Inflammatory foods
- Foods that trigger autoimmune disease
- Non-organic proteins
- Alcohol
- Caffeine

Pausing means just taking a break from certain things until your symptoms improve and you feel great. My plan for you is that you'll learn how to listen to your body, take a pause, think about your food choices, and make mindful decisions, rather than let impulse make them for you.

And I think you will love the results. Listen to what Annie told me about her experience: "I am 56 and in surgical menopause, in which my ovaries had to be removed. I have about 60 hot flashes a day, pretty much every 20 minutes during the day and about every hour at night. I started this program because my gynecologist/surgeon could offer me nothing for relief, short of antidepressants, which I emphatically refused.

"So, for 2½ months, I chose the Keto-Green Extreme program. I lost 15 pounds,

lots of inches, and had better skin. And not even one hot flash!"

I'm so happy for Annie and others like her. You can experience the same magic!

The 6-Day MenuPause Plans

The method by which you pause and restore peace, balance, harmony, energy, and health to your life is to follow one of my five plans and one or more of them at appropriate times during the year as needed.

Why five eating plans, and why six days?

Our dietary needs change as our hormones change. The nutrition you required at age 5 is much different from what you need at age 50. Maybe your slim, shapely figure is slipping away slowly as you enter menopause, or maybe you are like me and struggled with yo-yo dieting and excess weight most of your life. Weight gain during menopause is a hard and unignorable reality most of us have to brace ourselves for. But we can tackle it with the right *pause* strategies. Pausing from certain foods, and emphasizing other foods instead, has remarkable healing power, as you are about to learn.

Taking pauses can also help you break past the plateaus. We've all been there: you're a few months into a diet and the rate at which you were losing weight week after week has all of a sudden come to a halt. This is a signal to do something different.

Doing something different helps fight diet boredom, too. I don't know about you,

Understanding Menopause

Menopause is the time of life when we naturally stop having menstrual periods. It marks the end of our reproductive years. Because our periods can fluctuate during perimenopause (the phase when the ovaries start to produce less estrogen), you know you've truly hit menopause after you go 12 months without a period.

The average menopausal age is 51 in the United States, with perimenopause (the onset of hormonal fluctuation and a period of transition toward menopause) beginning from 5 or even 15 years before then. Sometimes, perimenopause can start as young as when we are in our 30s. You change a lot during these years. And, as you may remember from puberty, transitions can be awkward when your body and your mood frequently betray you.

For some women, menopause is not a life-shattering event. For others, it can be truly agonizing. In a survey by the American Association of Retired Persons, 84 percent of participating women said that menopausal symptoms interfered with their lives. My own symptoms were those that many of you have experienced: weight gain, brain fog, sleepless nights, hair loss, irritability, and more. I truly believed that if I just hung in there long enough, the symptoms would disappear. Unfortunately, that was not the case. They just seemed to go on forever.

Aside from the misery some of us have felt, we are not getting the help we should from our physicians. A 2013 Johns Hopkins University survey found that only 1 in 5 American obstetrics and gynecology residents had received formal training in menopause medicine. That's only 20 percent of gynecologists!

If they do pay attention to us, they give advice something like this: "Just ignore it; it's going to get better." Or, "You can take an antidepressant, which will help your hot flashes— but it's going to lower your sex drive and you might gain weight." Or, "Here, try this prescription for standard hormone replacement therapy, but it may increase your chances of getting blood clots, heart attacks, strokes, or breast cancer."

Whoa. Your body is already changing like crazy, and you surely don't want to burden it with more, and especially with pharmaceuticals that could potentially harm your well-being at the same time. (Full disclosure: Yes, I do believe in hormone replacement, as long as the hormones are bioidentical.)

Obviously, the options are not too fabulous. So, I'm not surprised that many women are casting about for more natural, safer approaches than pharmaceuticals—and nutrition is at the top of the list.

It works magic to fix our hormones, as I wrote about in my bestselling book *The Hormone Fix.* Nutrition and lifestyle rather than drugs are intimately involved in healing and regulating our master hormones—insulin, cortisol, and the most powerful of the three—the love, joy, and bonding hormone, oxytocin. When those three are working at peak function, our reproductive hormones, estrogen, progesterone, testosterone, and DHEA, are balanced throughout the menopausal journey.

Heal Your Gut in Three Days

Many women suffer gut problems during menopause. I've seen this with my patients and clients, and I know it all too well myself! I experienced years of suffering due to gut problems brought on mainly by sensitivity to dairy foods. In fact, even now, after being dairy-free for more than 15 years, when I eat something that contains dairy or whey, I get heavier (sometimes as much as 3 pounds) and bloated the next day.

The health of your gut is extremely important to the health of your entire body. Collectively called the *microbiome*, your gut houses trillions of healthy bacteria. It is their job to metabolize nutrients, produce vitamins, and detoxify harmful substances that make their way from the environment into your body. They also help power your brain, muscles, and immune system.

But as we age, our gut becomes challenged, and the healthy ratio of good bacteria to bad bacteria is imperiled. The immediate consequences are gas, bloating, acid reflux, constipation, and diarrhea. Although there are many potential causes of digestive problems, hormonal imbalance is one of the primary factors. Fortunately, this means that nutrition is generally the best place to begin to fix the issues. In many cases, gut problems can be eased by eating a more wholesome, fiber-rich diet and by drinking more water.

I bet I can read your mind right now: "I need relief now, Dr. Anna! I don't want to wait a long time for diet to fix my digestive issues."

Well, you'll be pleasantly surprised—maybe even overjoyed—to learn that you don't have to wait. You can boost the health of your microbiome within three days—without taking any medication—and alleviate your symptoms fast.

Proof of this comes from a 2013 Harvard University study. It found that gut bacteria can change just three days after making healthy dietary changes. The research team discovered that when people switch to an animal-based diet, the number of friendly gut bacteria that process protein increases. When they followed a plant-based diet, another type of good bacteria proliferates—the kind that processes starch and cellulose. This study demonstrates the amazing power of the foods we eat, and how fast those foods — both animal and plant foods—can heal us.

So, the solution to almost any gut problem is simple: build each meal around fiber-rich foods such as vegetables, beans, seeds, and nuts. Green plants are especially important because they are alkaline. Alkaline foods help heal the gut by supplying it with prebiotics—fiber-rich foods on which the friendly gut bacteria feed. Add healthy, organic protein foods for their own benefits. All these foods promote healthy gut bacteria, which in turn keep you happy and healthy and can add to the massive, diverse community of bacteria living and working within your digestive system. The plans in this book can help fast-track you toward great gut health.

but I'm easily bored by eating the same old thing day after day, no matter how good for me or how much it's changing my shape. I need to change things to stay on track. When we experience diet boredom, we might easily be tempted and stray from the diet. That won't happen with the *MenuPause* plans. You can try something new every six days, if you desire. Plus, since many of the recipes I offer in the pages to come work for more than one plan, you'll have a wide variety of recipes to keep you interested and on track.

I also feel that too often we just don't eat enough of the *right* foods. In doing so, we're missing out on a lot of healing and immune-boosting power. So, it helps from time to time to adjust what we eat and how we eat. We need to spread our wings, enlarge our food horizons, and get out of food ruts, if we're stuck in one.

As for six days, let's talk about this for a moment. Your marvelous body starts changing for the better within a short time after feeding it properly. Consider the results of what various clinical studies say about the rather quick effects of healthy food on your body within just a week:

After 15 minutes: If your first meal of the day is devoid of processed foods like white bread, sugary cereal, or doughnuts, but includes lean organic protein, fresh veggies, and healthy fats, you should feel energetic and mentally charged up after only one meal.

After 3 hours: The benefits keep on coming as that first healthy meal is absorbed. Your artery linings start to expand to increase blood flow to your tissues and organs.

After 6 hours: A day of nutritious eating perks up your HDL cholesterol in your blood and starts scrubbing the LDL cholesterol from your blood. That's why I refer to HDL—which technically stands for high density lipoprotein—as the "happy cholesterol." I call LDL the "lousy cholesterol."

After 12–16 hours: If you've eliminated sugar and cut way back on carbs, your body goes into a fat-burning state called ketosis.

After 24 hours: You might even be 1 or 2 pounds lighter, because you're still burning fat, along with flushing excess water and toxins from your body.

After 3 days: Once your body senses it is losing weight and getting good nutrition, its blood-related numbers (cholesterol, blood pressure, and blood sugar) start traveling in the right direction. As blood sugar and insulin start responding normally, you can expect a gradual decrease in hot flashes and night sweats, too. Other menopausal symptoms start their decline as well.

After 6–7 days: Blood levels of important anti-inflammatory and immune-boosting nutrients are higher. Your bowel is working better, and you should be around 5 pounds lighter. And maybe by the weekend, you can possibly fit into a smaller dress size!

Pretty amazing what can happen in six days, right? Don't you want to start feeling better right away? Of course, you do!

Which 6-Day Plan Is Right for You?

The answer depends on where you are right now, your health goals, and the symptoms you're experiencing. I'll get into the specifics of each plan later on, but for now, here's the thumbnail summary of each, as well as which symptoms are best managed through each plan:

The Keto-Green Extreme

This plan is based on three nutritional principles:

1. Ketosis. You eat in a ketogenic way: low in carbohydrates, moderate in protein, and high in healthy fat. This keeps your carbohydrate stores almost empty. Your body starts burning its own body fat for energy, helping you lose weight quickly and making you more insulin sensitive, which is key for healthy aging and for eliminating hot flashes.

2. Alkalinity. This plan strives to keep your urinary pH at an optimal "alkaline" level, which typically sits at 7 or above. A urine pH that is more alkaline than acidic is linked to lower rates of cancer, obesity and overweight, cardiovascular disease, metabolic syndrome, and other chronic diseases. Making sure you have an alkaline urine pH also helps ease any side effects of strict ketogenic eating.

   You can measure ketosis and alkalinity by using my special dual test strips (See the Resources section of this cookbook for information.)

3. Autoimmune Protection. I call this plan "extreme" because it pauses certain foods (even some considered "healthy") and replaces them with health-promoting, nutrient-dense foods that reduce inflammation and lower the symptoms of autoimmune diseases. Keto-Green Extreme allows *fewer* foods than my main Keto-Green nutritional plan.

This plan is best if you:

- Are experiencing these key symptoms of menopause: hot flashes, night sweats, brain fog, unexpected weight gain; and physical and mental tiredness.
- Need to lose weight steadily.
- Are "weight-loss resistant," meaning you have trouble dropping pounds.
- Have been diagnosed with hormonal imbalances.
- Have insulin resistance, prediabetes, or full-blown diabetes.
- Suffer from any type of autoimmune disease such as rheumatoid arthritis, lupus, inflammatory bowel disease (IBD), multiple sclerosis (MS), Type 1 diabetes, and psoriasis, among other conditions.

The Keto-Green Plant-Based Detox

This plan is 100 percent plant based. It swaps out animal foods for plant-based substitutes such as beans, legumes, tofu, and tempeh, while remaining high in alkaline vegetables.

This plan is best if you:

- Are a vegan or vegetarian.
- Want a break from animal products periodically, which I highly recommend.
- Are experiencing these symptoms of menopause: digestive problems (bloating, constipation, irritable bowel syndrome, and so forth), sleep disturbances, hot flashes, night sweats, and weight gain.
- Need to lose weight steadily.
- Have been diagnosed with hormonal imbalances or abnormal blood lipids (high triglycerides and high total cholesterol), or you've been told you're at risk for heart disease.
- Want to explore the plant-based lifestyle.

The Carbohydrate Pause

On this plan, you temporarily pause all carbohydrates and eat nothing but organic animal proteins. Before you roll your eyes, hear me out. True, this plan is not for everyone, but it is an effective way to smash past a weight-loss plateau and get the scale moving in a lower direction rapidly. It also quickly resolves bloating that you might experience from eating otherwise healthy but gas-producing roughage like cabbage or Brussels sprouts. What's more, people with autoimmune diseases have been known to benefit from plans like this one.

This plan is best if you:

- Want to stimulate fast weight loss at the start of your weight-loss efforts.
- Have hit a plateau after dropping pounds.
- Are "weight-loss resistant," meaning you have trouble dropping pounds.
- Have an autoimmune disease (a 100 percent protein diet has been shown to help with these conditions, too).
- Are insulin resistant.
- Experience menopause symptoms such as insulin resistance, sudden weight gain, hard-to-budge belly fat, cravings, sleep disturbances, frequent bloating, and brain fog.

Can My Guy Use These Plans, Too?

Absolutely! Weight gain, autoimmune problems, hormone imbalance, gut problems, and so forth are not the exclusive province of women.

Men go through "male menopause," or *andropause*, which is a decline in their hormones. As men age and transition through andropause, they will experience hormone changes that can impact their muscle, bone, brain, insulin resistance, and cardiovascular health—their zest for life and so much more.

We know, for example, that a man's testosterone peaks in his 20s and gradually declines about 1 percent a year after the age of 30. Testosterone is a sex hormone important to both men and women. It is essential for libido, arousal, and orgasm. In men it is also important relating to achieving an erection.

Additionally, a man may also start to produce and experience too much estrogen as he ages. Yes, estrogen. That can cause even more health symptoms and problems. His hormonal imbalances result in some of the same symptoms we experience:

- Increase in abdominal fat
- Brain fog and fatigue
- Night sweats
- Mood swings
- Increased risk of insulin resistance
- Bone loss and weakening
- Decreased muscle mass
- Moobs (very distressing male boobs)
- Decreased sex drive and performance

So, what's a man to do? Make the same nutritional and lifestyle changes (diet and keeping at a healthy weight are key) that I stress here—changes that naturally restore hormone balance.

Keith, a 57-year-old executive who started following the Keto-Green Extreme plan with 16 hours of intermittent fasting, texted me after three days to say that his cravings were gone after one month of staying "mostly 70 percent compliant" with the principles, he boasted his improved blood pressure, better energy, 15-pound weight loss, and defined abs. Of course, he also wanted to share about his improved sexual performance!

The road to health change can be bumpy, filled with the occasional potholes. But much like life's other journeys, the going is smoother when you have a loved one to share the trip with.

That's why it is so important to have a partner who not only shares your weight loss and health goals but can also take the journey with you. Many experts now say a supportive partner can make the difference between failure and success. And let's be honest; sexual function is really important, and keeping this aspect in a couple's lives may be the difference between divorce and a long, happy marriage.

The Keto-Green Cleanse

This is a liquid cleanse consisting of smoothies, juices, and broth that will restore and energize you at the cellular level.

Don't let that word "cleanse" scare you off. This is not a harsh detox that will leave you weak and shaky; rather, it's a gentle plan that will leave you strong, sculpted, and vitalized. It's not about deprivation—it's about restoration and renewal.

This plan is best if you:

- Are feeling burned out.
- Desire more energy.
- Want to lose weight, particularly belly fat.
- Struggle with food cravings.
- Need to detox your body after a period of eating too many processed and sugar-laden foods.
- Need to resolve specific menopause symptoms such as fatigue, joint pain, brain fog, constipation, and skin problems such as adult acne.
- Want to fast for spiritual growth.

The Carbohydrate Modification Plan

This is the most liberal of the five plans and it allows for the addition of healthy but gluten-free carbohydrates in your diet—as tolerated. Examples include higher-starch vegetables such as sweet potatoes, root vegetables, and legumes; and grains like quinoa, brown rice, and gluten-free oatmeal. There is more "feasting" on this plan, yet it is highly alkalizing and an excellent way to boost your immune health.

This plan is best if you:

- Have reached your desired weight and need to transition to a maintenance plan.
- Desire a more broad-based eating plan.
- Desire to keep hormones in balance, preventing the major symptoms of menopause, such as hot flashes, night sweats, sleep disturbances, fatigue, irritability and anxiety, depression, and memory problems.
- Are not carbohydrate sensitive (meaning carbs do not cause cravings or unexpected weight gain).
- Are gluten intolerant.
- Want to enjoy feasting (less rigid eating).
- Are training for a high-intensity athletic event and require a higher carb intake to fuel your training and competition.

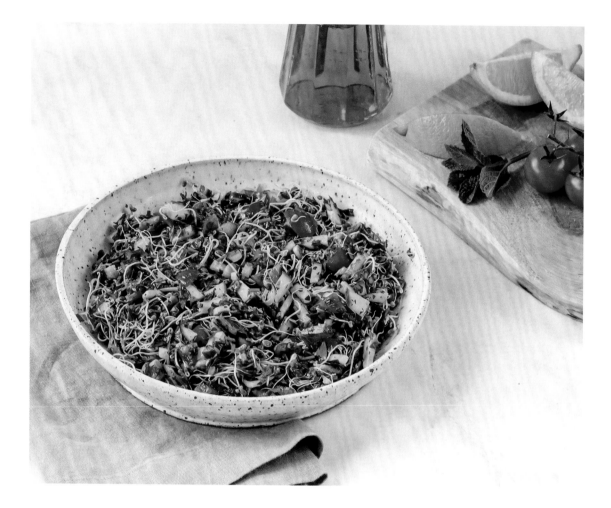

There you have it: the essence of *MenuPause*, supported by delicious foods and meals, all medically proven. And by the way, *you can try all these plans; you don't have to stay on just one.*

So, hang in there! Menopause doesn't mean the end of "normal" life. The way I look at it, it's an opportunity to optimize our habits—especially diet—so that we can happily and healthily live the lives we choose. The *MenuPause* recipes, and the extra resources I have for you (dranna.com/menupause-extras), will help you get there and be healthier and happier all the way around.

Above: Dr. Anna's Keto-Green Tabbouleh, page 182

Menopause Around the World: Asia

Japan gives us a beautiful example of a different attitude toward menopause—and a different experience of it, too. Japanese women tend to view menopause as their "second spring," a time of renewal. They worry even less about hot flashes and night sweats because they get them less frequently. There's a very good reason for that: their diet.

Many experts have suggested that menopause is much easier for Asian women than for Westerners because Asian women follow traditional, mostly plant-based diets. It is well documented that Western women eat much more meat, and about four times as much saturated fat, as women on traditional Asian plant-based diets, and only one-fourth to one-half the fiber that Asian women eat.

Plus, Japanese women do not consider menopause to be a sign of middle age; rather, they see it as a natural process. Their word for menopause is translated loosely as "renewal and regeneration." I believe that when you develop a positive mindset, including with a perspective like this, it changes your physiology to greater physical well-being and good health. Until recently, there was no word for "hot flash" in Japanese, and only about 25 percent of Japanese women even experience hot flashes!

For a taste of Asian-inspired *MenuPause* recipes, try Asian Zoodle Pad Thai (page 150), Keto-Green Tom Kha Gai (page 143), Miso-Ginger Zoodle Ramen (page 187), and Ginger-Soy Shredded Beef (page 224).

CHAPTER 2

How *MenuPause* Heals Your Body

The five *MenuPause* plans in this book work because they rely on food as our number-one remedy. I discovered the connection between food and menopause years ago, as I searched for answers to my own health issues that seemed beyond the conventional medical approach to healing.

It was during this same time that I realized I also had to take the biblical proverb "Physician, heal thyself" to heart. I needed to get well, feel better, and be stronger before I could help other women. My worldwide journey of study and research taught me that the help is not only in a medical prescription or pharmaceuticals—not by a long shot. I know that prescription medicines and surgery are sometimes necessary, but I've found that the best medicine to heal disease is found in lifestyle and in food— what we eat and what we don't eat.

As I mentioned earlier, other cultures seem to take this to heart more than ours in the United States, and their collective health shows it. They seem to intuitively know that it takes more than hormones to heal hormones. So, just remember: what you put on the end of your fork can be more curative than what you'll find at the bottom of a pill bottle.

The Food Fix

Food acts like a natural protector against disease in general, and it delivers menopause relief specifically. For example, nutritious, healing food:

Fights Inflammation. When you cut your finger, the redness and swelling at the wound are signs of inflammation. This short-term type of inflammation, known as acute inflammation, is beneficial because it means your immune system is responding to the injury and to intruders, such as bacteria, so as to heal your body. As your finger heals, the redness and swelling abate; the inflammatory response calms down. In this instance, your immune system detects that the short-term crisis that was your cut finger no longer requires a five-alarm response.

With chronic inflammation, however, your immune system fails to calm down. Instead, it releases a continual stream of inflammatory substances that negatively affect nearly every tissue, hormone, and

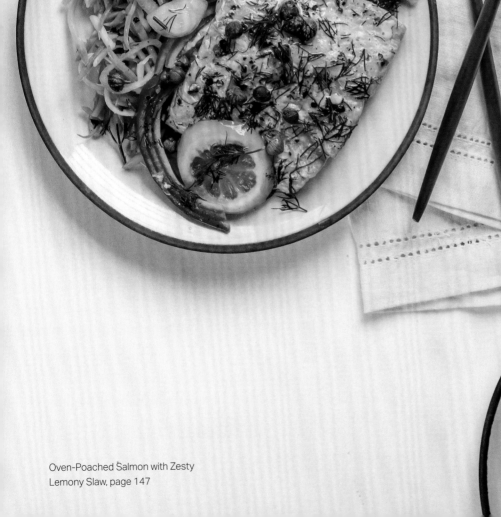

Oven-Poached Salmon with Zesty
Lemony Slaw, page 147

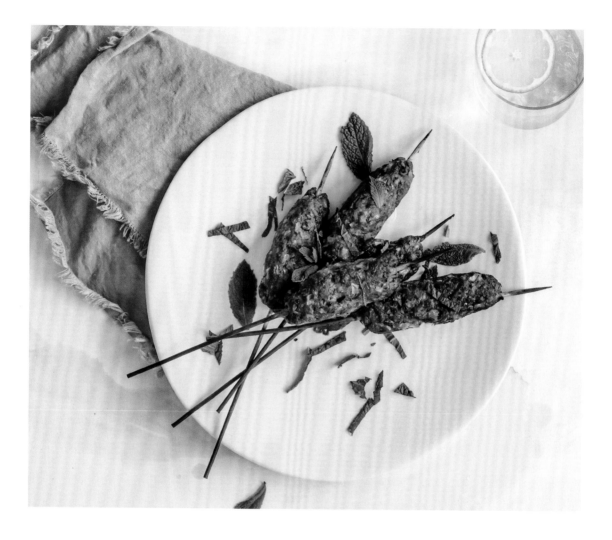

cell in your body. Chronic, unresolved inflammation is at the root of most diseases, so it needs to be tamed.

As you enter menopause, a sudden drop in your hormone levels can cause inflammation to rage throughout your body. This can be further compounded by menopausal weight gain. Fat tissue is known to release inflammatory agents that can increase your risk of diabetes, cardiovascular disease, and cancer.

In my programs, I have seen how dietary changes can dramatically reduce inflammation. In particular, women following my dietary recommendations have reported less joint pain, less menstrual discomfort, fewer mood swings, and reduced chronic pain due to inflammation (especially chronic back pain).

Says Lisa B.: "I've been a vegan for the

Above: Kafta Kabobs, page 210

past several years, so I chose to try the Keto-Green Plant-Based Detox. Choosing this plan has been huge on my emotional, mental, and physical health. Furthermore, I have even noticed changes in my marriage because of my hormones getting back in balance. I am less irritable and more happy on a daily basis. My goal of losing 16 pounds has turned into 27 pounds lost, and my husband has lost 20 pounds."

Balances Hormones. These chemical messengers impact every part of your health, from your energy and cognitive abilities to your body weight and sex drive. Our body relies on a delicate balance of reproductive hormones—estrogen, progesterone, testosterone, and DHEA—to function in a healthy way.

Hormonal imbalances, however, occur as we head into menopause and during perimenopause. These imbalances manifest as different issues in our body—headaches, aches and pains, menstrual irregularities, weight gain and bloating, as well as vaginal dryness, weakening pelvic floor muscles, incontinence, and decreased arousal.

Food is our white knight! We seldom make the connection between what we eat and how it affects our hormones, but food is our number-one hormone regulator!

Food does the following:

- Supplies the building materials to make hormones
- Increases the levels of certain hormones like insulin and changes the way estrogen and other female sex hormones are metabolized
- Elevates oxytocin (a major feel-good

hormone) and modulates cortisol (another major hormone)
- Stimulates the release of testosterone, important for your health as you get older

When you keep your diet on the alkaline side with lots of green vegetables and cruciferous veggies (like broccoli and cauliflower), your body begins to eliminate excess estrogen from your body and keeps the crazy feelings at bay (super important!).

Resolves Insulin Resistance. Initiated by a diet high in sugar and processed foods, and snacking, insulin resistance occurs when energy-yielding glucose (blood sugar) can't get into cells the way it normally would. As a result, it is eventually stored as fat.

Insulin resistance lurks beneath many of the most common symptoms you experience during menopause: hot flashes, fatigue, difficulty concentrating, and weight gain. All these point to insulin resistance, but we often don't make the connection because no one has told us!

My nutritional recommendations help regulate insulin and reverse insulin resistance in one important way: by restoring your body to an insulin-sensitive state and banishing menopause symptoms.

Builds Cellular Health. Great health starts at the cellular level. The nutrients your body absorbs from the food you eat can either build up or break down your body's health at a cellular level. Almost 2 trillion new cells are born in the body on a daily basis, and by choosing to eat the right foods, you are supporting the growth of those cells, ensuring their healthy life

Menopause Around the World: The Middle East

The Middle East region consists of 20 countries that extend from the Arabian Gulf to the Mediterranean Sea. I'm partially of Middle Eastern descent, so I grew up eating a lot of this amazing cuisine.

While writing this cookbook, I came across research called the Women's Cultural Wisdom Study. The researchers gave a questionnaire to 1,010 women in Iran and Japan, and found that in these cultures, women anticipated the arrival of menopause positively, reported fewer symptoms typically associated with menopause, and the symptoms they did experience were less severe. The diets of both these groups include lots of legumes with weak phytoestrogenic activity (chickpeas in Iran and soybeans in Japan). The researchers made a correlation between the intake of these legumes and the fact that these women had very few menopausal complaints. The study concluded by suggesting that American women should eat more chickpeas!

I can't say I was surprised by these results. Chickpeas are certainly an international superfood. For background, chickpeas are one of the most popular and widely used legumes in the Middle Eastern diet (they're called garbanzo beans in Hispanic cooking and ceci beans in Italian).

Their health benefits top the charts. They help control insulin and blood sugar. This is good for women with severe hot flashes. Chickpeas also ease digestive troubles because they are high in fiber, especially a soluble fiber called raffinose. The friendly bacteria in your gut dismantle this fiber so that your colon can digest it slowly and keep things moving.

Because they have calcium, magnesium, and fiber, chickpeas give you stronger bones, too. They also contain choline, a nutrient that helps make important chemicals for improving memory and mood—a benefit much needed when you're feeling brain foggy or anxious and irritable for no apparent reason.

So, chickpeas? Yes. Take a lesson from Middle Eastern cuisine and make them part of your diet. I like to substitute them for animal protein, and there are many ways to make them, including one of my favorites, hummus.

Some *MenuPause* suggestions are Arabic Garden Salad (page 171), Golden Cabbage Chickpea Soup (page 180), Comforting Spinach and Chickpeas (page 189), Keto-Green Hummus (page 173), Shakshuka (page 256), and Kafta Kabobs (page 210).

Other Middle Eastern foods are superstars, too: leafy greens, lean meats, and many other legumes and veggies.

One caveat: if you have an autoimmune disease, you'll want to pause legumes. See my explanation on page 56.

cycle. Cells are the building blocks of all our organs and tissues and are the smallest living organisms in our bodies.

Healthy eating allows our cells to heal the parts of our bodies that have been damaged.

Strengthens Immune Health. The immune system is like an army that attacks disease-causing invaders. Prior to menopause, we have healthy levels of estrogen, progesterone, and DHEA, all of which bolster our immune function. But as the production of these hormones drops off during and after menopause, we lose this protection.

Certain menopause symptoms can also undermine the immune system. For example, quality sleep is vital for a robust immune response, but menopause often brings on insomnia or other sleep disturbances that can prevent a good night's sleep.

Fatigue also stands in the way of regular physical activity, which can provide a boost to the immune system. Low libido and vaginal dryness can interfere with sex during menopause. Not having sex robs you of the immune and oxytocin boost that sexual activity affords you. Plus, struggling with menopause symptoms like hair loss, mood changes, weight gain, memory loss, and hot flashes is no walk in the park. They're stressful conditions, and high levels of the stress hormone cortisol will weaken your immune response.

Food to the rescue again! Fortunately, there's nothing more powerful than whole, natural foods to recharge your immune system and protect your body from menopause aggravations and illness.

Switches on Healthy Genes. Food holds information that communicates to our genes. In fact, scientists have learned that food "talks" to our DNA, switching on or off the genes that lead to health or disease. A good example are the omega-3 fats found in fish. They switch off genes that tell your body to release highly inflammatory substances. Amazing, right? What you eat programs your body with messages of health or illness.

So, yes, food is medicine!

Of course, that's not to say all food is medicine. The food you eat to help you breeze through menopause has to be whole, natural, and nutrient dense. Look at it this way: if you can pick it, peel it, fish it, hunt it, milk it, or grow it, you can eat it for menopause relief.

CHAPTER 3

6 Days to Menopausal Weight Loss, Energy, and Feeling Great

There is absolutely no question that the symptoms you're experiencing are annoying, painful, depressing—and for sure, they're upending your quality of life. As frustrating as hot flashes, night sweats, joint pain, and other complaints are, there is one symptom that affects all the others: menopausal weight gain. It is the one change that bothers most of us. I know it bothered me, even more than my brain fog, irritability, and moodiness.

What is so frustrating about menopausal weight gain is that it is stubborn. You might be following a healthy diet, cutting back on processed foods, but you're still gaining.

There is something else you should know about this symptom: if you're overweight or obese, or getting there, you may suffer more severe hot flashes, night sweats, and other symptoms than your slimmer peers!

In a Brazilian study, researchers compared menopause symptoms for women at a healthy weight to women who were either overweight or obese, and they found that three symptoms got progressively worse as women's size increased: hot flashes and night sweats, muscle and joint problems, and bladder issues.

As a doctor, I have observed this in patients. But I know that if we can tackle and resolve weight gain, other symptoms will diminish and we will be far healthier for it. So here, I want to spend a little time with you, talking about what I call the "worst menopausal symptom."

We want to relieve symptoms, not make them worse, right? So, weight control is absolutely essential to our well-being.

Opposite: Keto-Green Nachos, page 260

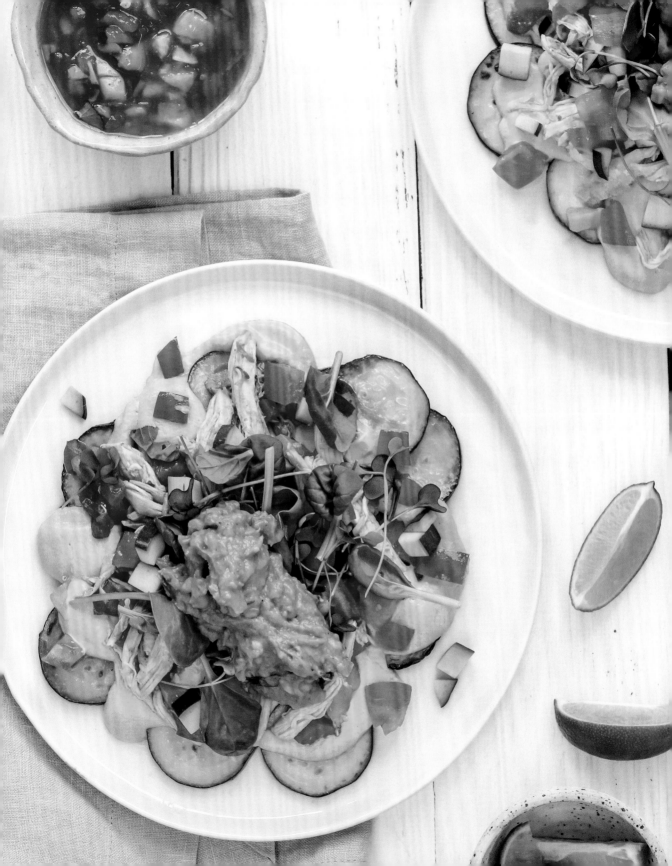

Why Do We Gain Weight at Menopause?

There are actually several reasons, all of which we can resolve. Take a look:

Estrogen Imbalance

The main culprit is reduced estrogen levels. Estrogen directs your body to store fat in certain places, like your hips or belly. As you inch toward menopause, it is the ups and downs (mostly downs) that do the most damage to your weight.

An estrogen shortfall leads to metabolic problems, which in turn plays havoc with how your body handles fat. As estrogen levels fall off, your body stores less subcutaneous fat (the pinchable stuff right under the skin) but begins to store it viscerally, meaning around abdominal organs.

Visceral fat is the dangerous kind of fat that leads to insulin resistance, diabetes, heart disease, and inflammatory diseases. On the bright side, it is easier to shed visceral fat with diet and exercise than subcutaneous fat.

Low estrogen levels also adversely affect hormones that control appetite and fullness, namely leptin and neuropeptide Y. A six-week animal study at Oregon Health and Science University showed that an imbalance of these hormones caused a 67 percent *increase* in food intake! And that naturally resulted in rapid weight gain, an average increase of about 5 percent in the six weeks.

Losing estrogen also impedes an activity in the body called *gluconeogenesis*. This is the process by which glucose is synthesized from non-carbohydrate sources. Very simply put, it is the conversion of protein or fat to sugar for the body to use as fuel. When this process slows down, less glucose is available to the brain for energy, and this results in brain fog, mental fatigue, and forgetfulness. In women, I've seen how all this can indirectly affect weight control in a psychological way. You don't even feel like putting forth the effort because you're so mentally tired.

A condition called *estrogen dominance* is another usual suspect. This refers to the fact that when menopausal changes ride into town, and we don't adjust our diets and lifestyle to suit these changes, our fat cells start storing excess estrogen from our diet and unnatural hormone-agents ("obesogens") in the environment. When this happens, there is more estrogen stored in our fat cells and this "dominates" our internal environment. Estrogen becomes the dominant hormone, interfering with the liver's ability to clear the excess. All this impacts other hormones. Weight gain is the result.

Another huge cause of estrogen dominance is plummeting levels of pro-gesterone. Yes, this decline is a natural part of aging, but it worsens in times of stress, both chronic and acute (see opposite page).

Low Vitamin D Levels

Insufficient estrogen levels may cause low vitamin D levels, which increases fat storage. Vitamin D is a fat-soluble vitamin that is produced in the skin with the help of sunlight and estrogen. Therefore, during menopause, many women are at risk of low vitamin D levels.

Because vitamin D is now recognized as a hormone, a short supply has negative effects. When vitamin D is low, hot flashes increase and memory loss and brain fog become worse. Vitamin D is such a powerful hormone for women to monitor in menopause because it is also implicated in so many other functions, from immunity to sleep quality. Ask your physician to test your vitamin D levels annually. Also, you can get a vitamin D boost from foods such as fatty fish, cod liver oil, egg yolks, and mushrooms. Supplementing with vitamin D3 (the most absorbable) is important as well. For self-testing options, see the Resources section of this book and dranna.com/menupause-extras.

Muscle Loss

We also lose calorie-burning muscle as we get older. Muscle is a metabolically active tissue that burns calories even when at rest, so you definitely do not want to lose it. Losing muscle leads to a complete deceleration in your metabolism. When this drop in metabolism is accompanied by the other changes I've described, extra pounds creep up on you. You can combat all this with resistance training, backed by adequate protein intake. Restore both your metabolism and your hormone balance in order to prevent weight gain.

Stress

Stress is a huge reason for weight gain during the menopausal years. The body purposely packs away some extra fat in times of internal or external stress as part of its survival mechanism. Along comes menopause, a time when we are grappling with other midlife challenges both personal and professional—retirement or more job responsibilities, financial worries, concerns over aging, struggles with kids or an empty nest, or caregiving our elderly parents—and all the resultant stress. Piled on top of these stresses is the stress that accompanies our other menopause issues (hello hot flashes!).

When your body is assaulted by stress, it churns out more adrenaline and cortisol. Adrenaline prompts a fight-or-flight response from your body, while cortisol mobilizes glucose for energy to defend yourself against the stressor. It also prods the body to store extra fat. This uptick of hormones can also stimulate you to eat more and endure cravings—more turns in an already vicious cycle!

Stress often jeopardizes your sleep, another factor that contributes to weight gain. Lack of sleep throws off the balance of leptin and ghrelin levels, the chemicals that control your appetite.

But diet can soften the hormonal havoc brought on by stress. One woman I've worked with, Andrea, put it this way: "Major life stress hit me a few years ago, which messed up my hormones, mainly cortisol. I was miserable emotionally and physically. I no longer recognized the girl in the mirror anymore. I then made the decision to take care of myself, and the payoff has been life changing. As of Thanksgiving 2020, I have lost about 75 pounds. I am thankful for the people in my life, but I am most thankful for the self-care and love I have poured into my life."

Understanding Other Health Risks

Yes, menopausal weight gain worsens our day-to-day symptoms, but it also increases our risk for some health-crushing illnesses. We're rarely told this by the medical establishment, and that's not only sad but also scary. Awareness is the beginning of healing, so I want you to know the serious downsides of menopausal weight gain.

Cancer Risk

Being overweight or obese is a risk factor for breast, endometrial, and uterine cancers. The reason is that fat tissue churns out excess estrogen, which has a negative estrogenic effect on the body that differs from naturally occurring levels of the hormone. A woman with a weight problem is constantly overexposed to estrogen, which is responsible for high cancer risk.

Higher body fat also poses an independent risk for complications such as kidney failure, liver disease, sleep apnea, pulmonary distress, and sexual dysfunction.

Diabetes and Heart Disease

If you put on weight at menopause, remember that fat gets distributed around your waist—a situation that increases your risk of Type 2 diabetes and heart disease.

As weight increases with menopause, glucose and insulin levels can also increase. This is the reason menopausal women also frequently have higher fasting insulin levels and insulin resistance, which drive weight gain, increase heart disease risk, and are the root causes of hot flashes.

Falls

Older obese women have a higher risk for falling, relative to women with a healthy weight, especially if excess fat accumulates around the waist. This weight affects the stability of your center of gravity, and therefore increases the incidence of fall-related injuries.

In the Global Longitudinal Study of Osteoporosis in Women (GLOW), researchers found that obesity, in contrast to widespread belief, is not protective against fracture but, rather, is responsible for certain fractures, mainly in the ankle and upper leg.

I mention this risk because fractures will affect your mobility and interfere with your ability to exercise. Physical activity is

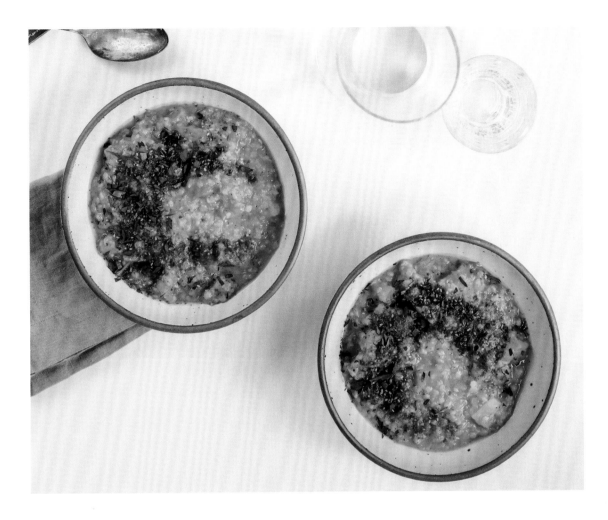

vital for offsetting menopausal muscle loss and your ability to lose weight. You want to avoid fractures at all costs!

Urinary Incontinence

It's not life-threatening, but urinary incontinence surely is both aggravating and embarrassing. Lack of bladder control is worsened by obesity. A 2018 study found that being overweight increased the risk of urinary incontinence for young and middle-aged women by 35 percent; obesity almost doubles the risk at 95 percent. The findings of this study are important because those with urinary incontinence when younger are more likely to have worse symptoms when they are older. Urinary incontinence should not be considered a normal part of aging, and it can be treated, even cured.

Above: Red Lentil and Squash Soup, page 178

Psychological Health

When you're dealing with weight issues, there's a psychological downside. Believe me, I know and I understand. When I was 80 pounds overweight, I'd get depressed and anxious—all stemming mostly from a poor body image. I just didn't like the way I looked. In some women, a poor body image leads to emotional overeating, then more pounds pile on and a vicious cycle ensues.

There's a physical issue that affects your psychological health, too. Obesity and overweight can cause problems in the gut. I'm referring to *dysbiosis*, a condition that alters levels of the feel-good neurotransmitter serotonin, most of which is produced in the gut. This situation disrupts even your willpower and positivity. You feel like you have little control over your body, your diet, your health.

Hope with MenuPause

Although the risk of weight gain as a menopausal woman is high, this does *not* mean that getting heavier is your destiny. It *does* mean that you may have to work more diligently to stop or keep your weight within a healthy range. If you can keep a healthy weight, or at least offset any weight gain, then you can minimize symptoms and unnecessary health risks, plus you will naturally create the willpower to stay with this for life.

Again, the hope lies in food. Food is a tool for weight loss. It helps your body burn fat—including menopausal weight gain—in many different ways. Some foods, for example, are high in a hormone called *adiponectin*. It acts in the brain to help you drop pounds and protect against gaining belly fat. It also fights weight-loss plateaus and promotes the use of fat for energy. Foods like avocados and olives, spices like turmeric, and fibrous veggies all raise levels of adiponectin in the body.

A classic fat-burner is protein. Studies suggest that high-protein foods require your body to burn a greater number of calories to digest them, compared with lower-protein foods. What's more, protein protects calorie-burning muscle tissue, keeping your metabolism high.

Certain foods act as natural appetite suppressants, too, especially protein, dietary fats, and high-fiber plant foods.

Plus, when you pause in consuming certain items such as carbohydrates and inflammatory foods, you put your body into a steady state of fat-burning.

So, yes: you can eat to lose!

MenuPause Around the World: The Mayan Culture

Contrary to what many think, the Mayan culture is alive and well. And Mayan women are special beneficiaries! Researchers have interviewed Mayan women in the rural regions of Guatemala and in Chichimilá, in the Yucatán Peninsula of Mexico, regarding their health and, in particular, about menopause. It turns out that these rural Mayan women hardly experience any traditional menopausal symptoms such as hot flashes, mood swings, and insomnia.

Plus, the women in Chichimilá, like the Japanese, seem to avoid osteoporosis. Although their estrogen levels gradually fall off at menopause, just like ours, and they lose bone mineral density, as we do, there is no clinical evidence of an increase in bone fractures or osteoporosis.

These women also have a positive mindset about getting older. What I find uplifting is that Mayan women, regardless of having symptoms or not, look forward to menopause and their newfound freedom and status.

Naturally, I wondered what their secret is for their good health and positivity. Again, diet emerges front and center. The Mayans have an all-natural, herb-based diet. Like the traditional Japanese diet, it is extremely low in animal products and low in fat in general.

For some delicious Mayan-like *MenuPause* recipes, try the following: Tomato Salad (page 172), Mexican Mushrooms (page 167), Keto-Green Nachos (page 260), and Red Lentil and Squash Soup (page 178).

PART 2

The 6-Day *MenuPause* Plans

Keto-Green Tom Kha Gai, page 145

CHAPTER 4

Keto-Green Extreme

In my other books, *The Hormone Fix* and *Keto-Green 16*, I introduced a way of eating that has helped thousands of women lose dangerous and menopause symptom-exacerbating weight: the Keto-Green protocol. Keto-Green eating combines ketogenic nutrition and alkaline eating, and it is a fantastically efficient and delicious way to reduce your symptoms and balance your hormones.

Get on This Plan If You:

- Have major symptoms of menopause: hot flashes, night sweats, brain fog, unexpected weight gain, and physical and mental tiredness.
- Need to lose weight steadily.
- Are "weight-loss resistant," meaning you have trouble dropping pounds.
- Have been diagnosed with hormonal imbalances.
- Have insulin resistance, prediabetes, or full-blown diabetes.
- Suffer from any type of autoimmune disease.

I love getting feedback from women who follow this plan. When I hear "My hot flashes are gone" or "No more skin flare-ups" or "I can finally sleep" or "I've got my figure back" and other success stories, I get really excited! Especially because the healing is based on diet, NOT on taking prescription drugs or other symptom-masking medical interventions.

That said, there are many women who tell me that the number on their scales won't budge after awhile, despite their best efforts at dropping pounds, and they've hit a plateau or stall. They've been successful at following my regular Keto-Green eating protocol, and are feeling better, but they are having trouble with weight—that big, dangerous symptom that affects so many aspects of physical and mental health related to menopause and afterward. In these instances, I always suspect a frustrating syndrome called *weight-loss resistance*. It is largely due to inflammation inflicting damage at the cellular level, particularly to the cell membranes. This damage makes it extremely difficult to trim your weight no matter how valiant your efforts. In these instances, the 6-day Keto-Green Extreme plan is in order!

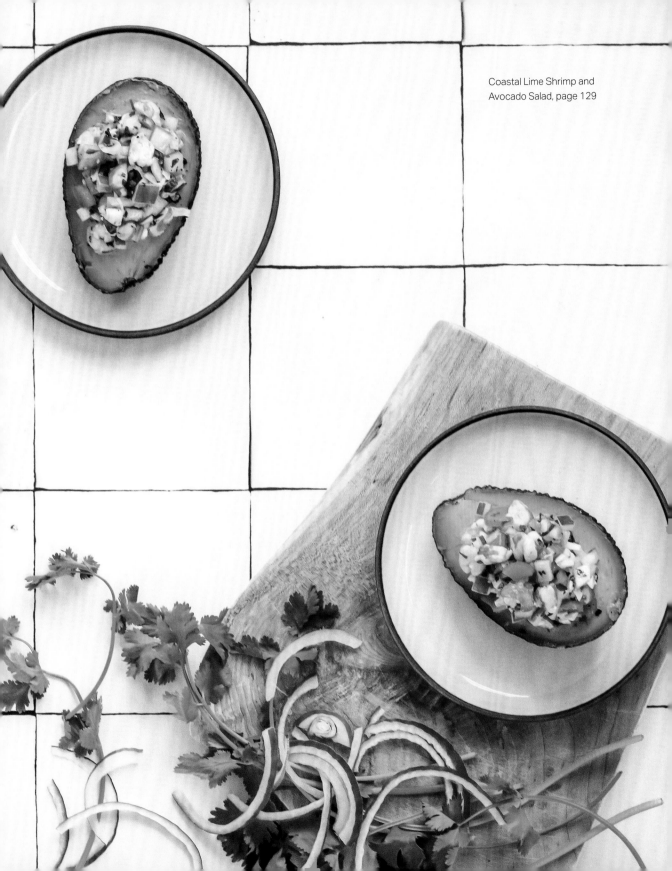

Coastal Lime Shrimp and
Avocado Salad, page 129

Understanding Weight-Loss Resistance

With weight-loss resistance, the inflammation is related mostly to auto-immune disease. Autoimmune disease is not rare: approximately 40 million Americans suffer from at least one autoimmune condition. And autoimmune disease causes inflammation that brings on weight gain.

Autoimmune conditions include rheumatoid arthritis (RA), Hashimoto's thyroiditis (hypothyroidism), multiple sclerosis (MS), Crohn's disease, colitis, celiac disease, Type 1 diabetes (T1DM), and lupus, among many others. Although these diseases affect different parts of the body, they all have one thing in common: they cause the body to attack itself, triggering inflammation.

Inflammation works its way right down to your fat cells. When they become inflamed, they can't release stored fat. Fat gets locked inside the cells, and it's difficult to liberate it.

If this happens to you, your body has a harder time maintaining your optimal weight range. It can be a vicious cycle, because the more weight you gain, the more inflamed your body becomes. On top of that, the more painful it can be to perform daily movement, which you also need for weight control.

Here's where Keto-Green Extreme helps. It is a way to avoid foods that cause weight-loss resistance and instead select foods that will help your fat cells release fat, so you start dropping pounds once again.

The results can be uplifting and truly amazing. One of the women in my Keto-Green Facebook community, Mary D., is proof. She cut out all fruit, dairy, and nuts—foods that are commonly unfriendly if you're suffering from autoimmunity. Mary lost 9 pounds in seven days. I think that is a record!

So, with its specific list of healing foods, Keto-Green Extreme can help you soothe autoimmunity, control inflammation, and get your scale moving in the right direction again.

Keto-Green Extreme, Explained

The 6-day Keto-Green Extreme plan is what you might expect from its name: a more extreme and shorter-lasting version of my *Keto-Green 16* diet. It has specific benefits for women experiencing weight-loss resistance, autoimmune disorders, insulin resistance, and the common symptoms of menopause.

What makes it extreme is that it offers fewer food choices. For example, there are no nuts or seeds on the plan, and nightshade vegetables such as tomatoes and eggplants are not allowed. Nor are beans and legumes. Normally, these foods are considered super-healthy, but for women with hard-to-resolve menopause issues, they are all wrong.

Keto-Green Extreme has three main parts that work in your favor.

Ketogenic Nutrition

Let's start with the "keto" part. This takes its name from the term *ketosis*—a metabolic state in which the body does not have enough glucose (sugar from carbohydrates) for energy, and therefore begins to burn fat. You lose weight as a result. In the process, your body produces ketone bodies. These can be measured in your urine and indicate whether or not you are burning fat.

Ketogenic eating requires that you keep your carb intake to 40 grams a day or less. As such, you must abstain from foods like rice, grains and cereals, potatoes, starchy vegetables, breads, pasta, sugar, most fruits, and dairy products.

Eliminating carbs is only part of the story, however. Because your body has a limited supply of glucose, it needs an alternative source of fuel. That fuel is fat—and lots of it. This plan is centered on a high intake of healthy, mostly plant-based fats—around 65 percent of your daily calories. You'll eat fats such as avocado, avocado oil, olive oil, coconut or MCT (medium-chain triglycerides) oil, and omega-3 fats from protein sources like salmon and other fatty fish.

Fat is so important to our hormones. For years, dietary advice spewed out the mantra that fat free is good, whereas all fat is bad. This is a dangerous lie. Fat is an important building block to produce and maintain proper hormone function, so if we're missing fat, problems arise simply because the body doesn't have the nutrients it needs to manufacture hormones.

The third key factor in keto nutrition is protein. You eat it in moderate proportions: about 25 percent of your daily calories. Protein is a highly "thermogenic" macronutrient, meaning that it raises body heat and thus increases metabolism and fat burning. Protein may even help you spot-reduce your tummy. In a number of studies, people who increased their intake of lean proteins to 25 to 30 percent of their total diet shed more belly fat than people who ate less protein.

This is so because protein rebalances

several appetite-regulating hormones. It lowers levels of the hunger hormone ghrelin, while it boosts the appetite-reducing hormones GLP-1 (glucagon-like peptide-1), peptide YY, and cholecystokinin. The result? Numerous studies have shown that if you increase your protein intake, you don't consume as many calories.

That lovely body-defining muscle of yours? Well, it begins to decrease during perimenopause and continues its slide unless you eat enough protein. Protein saves precious muscle from making its exit as we get older.

Protein choices on this plan are varied and include lean organic meats, poultry, eggs, wild-caught fish, and shellfish.

Alkalinity

Keto-Green Extreme emphasizes an important factor not present in the standard keto diet: alkalinity. An alkaline diet strives to keep your urinary pH at an optimal alkaline level, which typically sits at 7 or above.

An alkaline diet has also been shown to lower inflammation, decrease joint pain, and relieve menstrual discomfort. A urine pH that is more alkaline works to balance your hormones, gives you more energy, and helps you feel better overall.

With ketogenic nutrition paired with alkaline nutrition, you have the very best diet for women, with spectacular benefits. This approach:

- Boosts your metabolism and optimizes your hormones, allowing your body to efficiently burn fat for energy. Along with ketogenic nutrition, it trains your body to burn fat.

- Stabilizes blood sugar and makes you insulin sensitive, so you don't have to worry as much about high blood sugar, weight gain, and various menopausal symptoms—especially hot flashes, which are caused by insulin resistance.

- Tames hunger pangs—no more giving in to cravings.

- Detoxifies your body of pollutants, chemicals, and hormone disruptors that keep you from losing weight.

- Prevents the frequently reported side effects of standard keto diets: stomach upset, irritability, and a low-grade flu feeling (hence the nicknames "keto flu," and "keto craziness"!).

- Supports the health of practically every organ in your body, including your heart, brain, bones, sexual organs, gut, and skin.

To encourage alkalinity, concentrate on foods, herbs, and spices that make your body more alkaline. One of the most important food groups is green leafy vegetables, hence the "green" in Keto-Green Extreme. Think lettuce (all types); spinach; kale, dandelion greens; arugula; turnip, collard, beet greens, and mustard greens; and Swiss chard, among others. All these leafy greens keep your body in an alkaline state, plus they are superstars when it comes to detoxing your body. The veggies are also anti-inflammatory.

I also emphasize cruciferous vegetables for boosting alkalinity. These are basically your cabbage-family veggies such as broccoli, cabbage, cauliflower, and Brussels sprouts. They are so-named because they have "cross-shaped" flower petals.

I tagged these veggies for several of the *MenuPause* plans for a number of reasons. First, they contain indole-3-carbinol (I3C), a natural compound that stops the growth and expansion of fat cells. It works primarily by reducing a bad form of estrogen that can lead to fat accumulation and interfere with muscle development.

Second, cruciferous vegetables contain a natural ingredient called 3,3'-Diindolylmethane (DIM) that helps to destroy harmful synthetic estrogens in the body. These estrogens come from various sources, including gasoline fumes, plastics, medicines, pesticides, and perfumes—any product of petrochemical manufacturing.

Third, cruciferous veggies release sulfur-containing nutrients that help the liver detoxify and block cancer cell formation.

You will find that my recipes use lots of herbs and spices, as well as sea salt and, occasionally, sprouts. All these are highly alkalinizing, not to mention flavorful.

Another simple, powerful way to alkalinize your body is to include maca root in your diet. One of the stops on my healing journey was in the mountainous regions of the Peruvian Andes, where I learned about maca. I sampled it and began to drink it regularly. It restored my physical and mental energy. I felt more balanced and more alive than I had in a long time.

Eventually, I formulated my own product, Mighty Maca® Plus. It has been a long-term supplement for me and thousands of women who follow my programs and have seen great results. Visit dranna.com/menupause-extras to request a sample.

Maca root is a member of the radish family. It has a long, revered history of boosting hormone production and libido. After taking it, many women notice fewer PMS symptoms, increased fertility, improved skin, weight loss, energy, a higher sex drive, and more. Maca is also high in minerals and essential fatty acids, making it great for hormones. You will discover many recipes in this cookbook that use maca.

An alkaline diet also generally limits acidic foods like excess meat, cheese, grains, breads, pasta, sugar, artificial sweeteners, wheat products, processed carbohydrates, and sodas. The typical American diet is too high in these acid-producing foods. When your bodily fluids are too acidic, a situation known as *acidosis* is created. Acidosis occurs when your kidneys and lungs can't keep your body's pH in balance. Mineral levels are depleted, and chronic inflammation can set in.

Staying alkaline prevents these consequences. It also helps optimize the body's main hormonal players (insulin, cortisol, oxytocin). When these "master hormones" are balanced, many other hormones, such as estrogen and pro-gesterone, come into balance more quickly.

I recommend that you test your urine pH regularly, using test strips you can obtain at most pharmacies or at dranna.com/menupause-extras. Your urine pH goal should be in the 7 range in the morning. This normally takes a while to achieve, so be patient and stay the course. Knowing your pH is a simple and enlightening way to determine whether your physiology is measuring up or falling short.

Autoimmunity Protection

Here comes the "extreme" part of this plan—and the way by which you help reverse weight-loss resistance. It's designed to be a short-term protocol to reduce inflammation while healing autoimmune disease. Autoimmunity happens when your body's immune system starts attacking its own organs, tissues, and cells. Symptoms materialize slowly, with problems such as achy joints, fatigue, tummy troubles, and others.

But there's one symptom that many autoimmune diseases share: weight-loss resistance. Almost everyone with an auto-immune disorder has it affect their weight.

In autoimmunity, one of the causes of inflammation is a condition called "leaky gut." This simply means that your intestinal lining is more permeable than it should be. Normally, the gut lining absorbs nutrients from the food you've eaten and digested, and it blocks bacteria, wastes, and undigested food from entering your bloodstream. But with a leaky gut, gaps form in the intestinal walls and they allow food particles, wastes, bacteria, and toxins to escape into the bloodstream.

The body then identifies the leaked particles as foreign invaders and mounts an immune defense against them, leading to inflammation throughout your system, right down to the cellular level, including fat cells.

This entire scenario places an additional burden on your immune system, compromising its ability to fight off infections. The strain will also hyper-stimulate your immune system, and you're more likely to develop weight-loss resistance.

Nutritional research has identified foods that help or hurt autoimmune diseases. When you pause consuming certain foods and replace them with health-promoting, nutrient-dense foods, you can reduce inflammation and the symptoms of autoimmune diseases.

What You'll Eat on Keto-Green Extreme

When purchasing these foods, try to choose organic versions, if possible. In the case of protein, your choices should be grass-fed (meat), organic and pasture-raised (poultry), and wild-caught (fish). For more information, see page 79.

Vegetables

Artichokes
*Arugula
Asparagus
*Avocados (technically a fruit)
*Beet greens
Bok choy
Broccoli
Brussels sprouts
Cabbage
Carrots
Cauliflower
*Chard
*Cilantro
*Collard greens
Cucumbers
*Dandelion greens
*Endive
*Escarole
Fennel
Jicama
*Kale
Leeks
*Lettuce
*Maca
Mushrooms
*Mustard greens
Onions
*Parsley
*Radicchio
Radishes
*Spinach
Squash, summer
*Turnip greens
*Watercress
*Zucchini

*These veggies are highly alkalinizing.

Fruits (optional, but no more than one serving a day since fruits are generally high in carbohydrates)

Apples
Apricots
Berries
Cherries
Lemons
Limes
Mangos
Papaya
Peaches
Pears
Pineapple

Proteins

Beef
Bison
Bone broth
Chicken
Duck
Fish and shellfish
Lamb
Organ meats
Pork
Turkey
Venison

Fats

Avocado oil
*Avocados
Coconut oil
Ghee
MCT oil
Olive oil

* Avocado is highly alkalinizing.

Herbs and Spices

Basil
Bay leaf
Chives
Cinnamon
Dill
Garlic (technically a vegetable)
Ginger
Mint
Peppermint
Rosemary
Saffron
Sage
Thyme
Turmeric

Additional Foods (in moderation—up to 1 cup daily)

Nut milks, almond, cashew, and coconut
Dr. Anna's Keto-Green Shake (1 to 2 scoops daily)

What You'll Pause on Keto-Green Extreme

Gluten and Grains

If you have an autoimmune disease or are at risk for one, be aware that gluten, the protein in wheat that gives bread its airy volume, is highly inflammatory and should definitely be avoided. Grains that do not contain gluten can also be inflammatory in susceptible people. Pause the following:

Amaranth	Quinoa
Barley	Rice
Buckwheat	Rye
Bulger	Sorghum
Corn	Spelt
Millet	Wheat
Oats	

Protein

Eggs

Dairy

Butter	Ghee (clarified
Cheese	butter)
Cream	Milk
	Yogurt

Legumes

Legumes contain inflammatory chemicals called lectins, which are plant proteins that bind to carbohydrates. Just like all living things, plants have evolved to survive. Because they can't run and therefore can't escape invaders, plants have developed chemicals to repel pests. One type of chemical is lectins. The problem with most lectins, however, is that they promote inflammation in our bodies. They can also increase the possibility of leaky gut, in two ways: first, by damaging the cells that line the gut; and second, by causing an inflammatory response once outside the gut. To avoid lectin damage on Keto-Green Extreme, pause these foods:

Black beans	Lentils
Chickpeas	Lima beans
Cocoa powder	Soybeans and
Fava beans	soybean
Kidney beans	products

Nightshades

Although these foods are rich sources of nutrients and serve as cuisine staples in many cultures, plants in the nightshade family contain a group of natural chemicals called alkaloids. They're often very bitter and function as a natural insect repellent. For those with autoimmune conditions, alkaloids can stimulate and exaggerate an immune response. They are believed to increase the immune response to proteins leaking out of the gut. On Keto-Green Extreme, pause these nightshades:

Eggplants	Potatoes
All red spices	Tomatillos
All peppers	Tomatoes

Nuts and Seeds

Although these foods are allowed on my regular Keto-Green plan, nuts and seeds are high in lectins, too. This is one of the main reasons why nuts and seeds are excluded in diets meant to heal autoimmune diseases. On Keto-Green Extreme, pause these foods:

Almonds	Cashews
Brazil nuts	Chia seeds

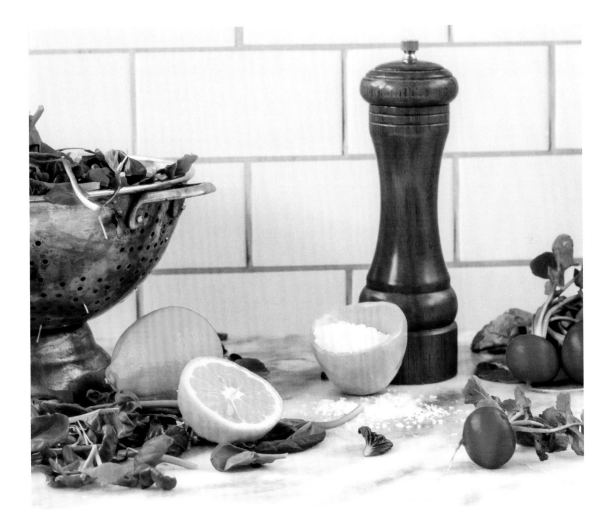

Coffee

Flax seeds

Hazelnuts

Hemp seeds

Pecans

Pine nuts

Pistachios

Pumpkin seeds

Sesame seeds

Sunflower seeds

Walnuts

Seed and Berry Spices

Allspice

Anise

Caraway

Celery seed

Cumin

Fennel seed

Nutmeg

Pepper

Poppy seed

Other Substances to Pause (These Are Highly Inflammatory)

Added sugar

All alcohol

Processed foods (aka "junk food")

The Keto-Green Extreme 6-Day Food Plan

Note: Each recipe makes two servings, with the exceptions of shakes and smoothies (which make 1 serving). So, feel free to enjoy leftovers for any meal.

For a downloadable menu plan with a graphic representation of the meals, go to dranna.com/menupause-extras.

Day 1

Breakfast
Good Morning Farmer's Breakfast Casserole OR
Dr. Anna's Basic Keto-Green Meal Replacement Shake

Lunch
Coastal Lime Shrimp and Avocado Salad

Dinner
Georgia Buffalo Shepherd's Pie AND Garlic-Roasted Asparagus

Day 2

Breakfast
Leftover Good Morning Farmer's Breakfast Casserole OR
Dr. Anna's Basic Keto-Green Meal Replacement Shake

Lunch
Asian Zoodle Pad Thai

Dinner
Fennel and Leek Pot Roast AND Rainbow Mediterranean Salad

Day 3

Breakfast
Smoked Salmon Breakfast Tower

Lunch
Dr. Anna's Cauliflower and Leek Soup

Dinner
Chicken and Bacon Cruciferous Stir-Fry AND Cauli Rice with Veggies

Day 4

Breakfast
Leftover Smoked Salmon Breakfast Tower OR
Extreme Green Smoothie

Lunch
Tuna and Celery Hand Salad OR Greek Keto-Green Salad

Dinner
Leftover Chicken and Bacon Cruciferous Stir-Fry AND Cauli Rice with Veggies OR Cabbage and Kale Bratwurst Skillet

Day 5

Breakfast
Avocado Veggie Toast OR
Dr. Anna's Basic Keto-Green Meal Replacement Shake

Lunch

Keto Green Tom Kha Gai OR

Warm Spinach/Kale Salad with Bacon with
 Basil-Thyme Vinaigrette

Dinner

Mom's Coq au Vin AND Roasted Brussels
 Sprouts with Radishes

Day 6

Breakfast

Extreme Green Smoothie

Lunch

Egg Roll Soup Bowl

Dinner

Oven-Poached Salmon with Zesty Lemony
 Slaw OR Lemony Broccoli OR

Halibut with Arugula Salad and Avocado
 Chimichurri

The DIY Meal Option

In addition to using the recipes, you can build your own meals by following a simple template:

Breakfast = 1 protein serving + 1 serving of permissible vegetables or fruit + 1 fat serving.

An example would be 2 ounces smoked salmon, 1 cup spinach or an herb-lettuce blend, and sliced ½ avocado drizzled with olive oil and sprinkled with sea salt.

Lunch = 1 protein serving + 1 to 2 servings of permissible vegetables + 1 to 2 fat servings.

An example would be 1 pan-fried ground beef patty + 1 to 2 cups spinach, kale, or beet greens sautéed in 1 tablespoon olive oil or coconut oil.

Dinner = 1 protein serving + 2 servings of permissible vegetables + 1 to 2 fat servings.

An example would be 1 baked chicken thigh or 6-ounce steak + mashed cauliflower + side salad with fresh greens tossed with 1 tablespoon olive oil, lemon juice, and garlic seasoning.

Your 6-Day Shopping List

You may not need to purchase all these items; you probably have many of them in your kitchen and pantry right now. Also, what you buy depends on which menu options you choose, or whether you DIY some of your meals. This shopping list is based on using all the recipes. It is designed for 2 people, so if you are cooking for 1, purchase only half of each item.

For a downloadable shopping list of this plan, go to dranna.com/menupause-extras.

Supplements and Staples to Have On Hand

Dr. Anna's Keto-Green or Keto-Alkaline Meal Replacement mix; or a good substitute protein powder formulated with a vegan protein such as pea or rice protein and containing less than 3 grams of sugar (per serving) and less than 10 grams of carbohydrate (per serving)

Mighty Maca Plus, 7.2-ounce container; or 1 (1-pound) bag maca root powder

Collagen powder, 1 (9.5-ounce) container

Coconut aminos, 1 (16-ounce) package

Nutritional yeast, 1 (5-ounce) package

MCT or coconut oil, 1 (16-ounce) bottle

Avocado oil, 1 (16-ounce) bottle

Extra-virgin olive oil, 1 (16-ounce) bottle

Ghee (clarified butter), 1 (13-ounce) jar

Apple cider vinegar, 1 quart

Balsamic vinegar (sugar-free), 1 (16-ounce) bottle

Red wine vinegar, 1 (16-ounce) bottle

White wine vinegar, 1 (16-ounce) bottle

Dry red wine, 1 (750 ml) bottle

Dijon mustard, 1 (8-ounce) jar

Garlic, minced, 1 (4-ounce) jar

Seasonings: sea salt, garlic powder, onion powder

Dried herbs: celery flakes, thyme or za'atar blend, oregano, bay leaves, Italian herbs, sumac

Produce—Fresh Vegetables

Spinach, 8-ounce bag

Baby spinach, 8-ounce bag

Arugula, 1 (16-ounce) bag

Romaine lettuce, 1 head

Kale, 3 (16-ounce) bags

Green cabbage, 2 small heads

Red cabbage, 1 small head

Brussels sprouts, 1 pound plus 1 package shaved Brussels sprouts

Broccoli, 2 small crowns

Broccoli slaw, 1 (16-ounce) bag

Cauliflower, 2 heads

Radishes, 1 bunch

Cucumbers, 4 Persian or 2 English

Celery, 1 bunch

Asparagus, 1 bunch

Carrots, 4 medium, 1 large

Zucchini, 1 large

Yellow onions, 2 small, 6 medium

Red onions

Shallots, 12 small, 1 medium, 1 large

Scallions, 1 large bunch

Leeks, 2

Garlic, 4 to 5 bulbs

Celeriac, 1 medium

Fennel, 2 bulbs
Bean sprouts, 1 (4-ounce) package
Baby bok choy, 4 bunches
Fresh ginger, 1 (2-inch) piece
Mushrooms, 1 (16-ounce) package
Shiitake mushrooms, 1 (16-ounce) package
Portobello mushrooms, 4

Produce—Fresh Herbs

Basil, 1 (.5-ounce) package or bunch
Cilantro, 1 bunch
Dill, 1 (.5-ounce) package or bunch
Kaffir lime leaves 1 (1-ounce) package
    (available from many online sources)
Lemongrass, 1 (.5-ounce) package
Mint, 1 (.5-ounce) package or bunch
Oregano, 1 (.5-ounce) package or bunch
Parsley, 1 bunch
Thyme, 1 (.5-ounce) package

Produce—Fresh Fruits

Avocados, 6 medium
Lemons, 10
Limes, 3

Protein Sources

Salmon, smoked, 1 (3-ounce) package,
    wild-caught
Salmon, 2 fillets (4 to 6 ounces each),
    wild-caught
Shrimp, jumbo, 12 ounces
Halibut, 2 fillet pieces (4 to 6 ounces each),
    wild-caught, or other firm-fleshed
    whitefish
Tuna, 2 (5-ounce) cans
Chicken breast, 1, with skin and bone
    (8 ounces)
Chicken cutlets, 8 ounces
Chicken thighs, boneless, skinless, 14 ounces
Chicken thighs, 2, with skin and bone
    (8 ounces total)
Chicken drumsticks, 2, with skin and bone
    (8 ounces total)
Beef chuck roast, boneless, 1 pound
    (preferably grass-fed)
Beef or bison, ground, 1 pound (preferably
    grass-fed)
Pork, ground, 8 ounces
Organic bratwurst, such as Organic Prairie,
    1 (12-ounce) package
Bacon (no-sugar), 8-ounce package

Non-Dairy Milks

Unsweetened almond milk, 1 quart
Full-fat unsweetened coconut milk,
    3 (14-ounce) cans

Other Items

AIP Rustic Bread Mix or Casabi Artisan
    Flatbread
Capers, 1 (3.5-ounce) jar
Kalamata olives, pitted, 1 (6.5-ounce) jar
    or can
Beef broth, 2 (32-ounce) packages
Chicken or vegetable broth, 3 (1-quart)
    packages
Cauliflower rice, frozen, 1 or 2 (10-ounce)
    packages
Blueberries, frozen, 1 (10-ounce) bag

Strategies for Success

1. Follow this plan exactly as written or substitute any meal with DIY meals you create based on the food lists.

2. You have the option of intermittent fasting on this plan. This type of fasting condenses your entire food intake to a specific window of time. A popular way to begin intermittent fasting is to have 16 hours of fasting and 8 hours of feeding, or 16:8. So, for example, if you have your last meal at 6:00 p.m., you wouldn't eat the next day until after 10:00 a.m. Intermittent fasting helps with weight loss, reduced inflammation, cellular renewal, detoxification, and other conditions.

    Alternatively, you may feel that you require only two meals daily within an 8-hour eating window, as having just two meals feels satisfying. This is an effective way to eat, because it encourages weight loss.

3. Test your urinary pH and ketones first thing in the morning (and periodically throughout the day whenever you go to the bathroom), with the goal of keeping your pH at or above 7.0. The pinker the strip, the higher your level of ketosis (fat-burning). Record everything in a journal. See the Resources section of this book, or go to dranna.com/menupause-extras for a downloadable journal page and how to order my strips.

4. Weigh yourself each morning so as to monitor whether you are becoming *less* weight-loss resistant.

5. Hydrate! Drink approximately half your ideal body weight in ounces of filtered water each day. But don't drink more than 4 ounces (½ cup) of fluids with any given meal, so that your digestive juices have time to do their work. My typical recommendation is to drink water up to 20 minutes before you eat, then have that 4 ounces of fluid with your meal, and wait one to two hours before drinking anything again.

6. Never overload your stomach. When you begin to feel full, stop eating.

7. Do not eat between meals and do not snack. Snacking can be destructive to your goals. It can cause insulin resistance, weight gain, hot flashes, and inflammation. You can add more healthy fats and oils to green leafy salads or enjoy a large cup of one of my bone broths (see pages 240–46).

8. On day 6, observe how you have been feeling, particularly with regard to common autoimmune symptoms such as fatigue, joint pain and swelling, digestive discomfort, resistant weight loss, or skin problems. If your improvements are minimal, resume the plan for another 6 days, or longer, and check your symptoms periodically. Once you feel improvements, switch to the 21-day Keto-Green Plan in *The Hormone Fix*, or transition to the Carbohydrate Modification Plan in this book.

Menopause Around the World: Rituals at Mealtime

Rituals are symbolic behaviors that are comforting in their repetition. Many cultures in the world practice rituals that are centered on food: the fasting and feasting that mark the holy days in Catholic, Muslim, and Jewish traditions; the gracious tea ceremonies in Asia (see page 94); or the harvest festivals that are celebrated everywhere from Kenya to Kentucky. According to archaeological studies, mealtime rituals have been important elements of human life for tens of thousands of years.

The benefits of rituals are many, both physical and psychological. For example, rituals are associated with the secretion of oxytocin in the brain. One of our master hormones, along with insulin and cortisol, oxytocin is responsible for bonding, and it is associated with empathy, trust, and relationship building. It also helps ease depression, anxiety, sexual dysfunction, anxiety, and gastrointestinal issues.

Rituals centered on meals have been described by researchers as "an underappreciated battleground to fight obesity." This is because studies have found that families—parents and children—who frequently dine together have healthier weights. As I've explained, proper weight is extremely important to maintaining great health, especially during menopause.

Other lines of evidence support the psychological benefits of food ritual, such as building social support and bolstering self-esteem.

The bottom line is this: mealtime rituals are important for a healthy menopause and a healthy life. So, how can you create eating rituals that will benefit your well-being? Here are four easy, no-fuss suggestions:

1. *Set a lovely table.* Use your favorite placemats and napkins, along with silverware. Use your best tableware, too. Have your children set the table—it is an important life skill and gets everyone involved. A beautifully set table is inviting and prepares everyone for the meal.
2. *Light candles.* I love candles because they cast a relaxing glow. One of the goals of any meal ritual is to relax and connect. Lighting candles is an easy way to accomplish this. Plus, they make every meal a special occasion.
3. *Bless your meal.* Saying grace or giving a blessing before eating acknowledges reverence, gratitude, and appreciation for the food and the nourishment it bestows. Your blessing could be as simple as: *May we be nourished, that we may nourish life.*
4. *Enjoy each other.* In my family, we take turns sharing the joys of our day. This gives us the chance to appreciate each other. Very important: avoid unnecessary conflicts or criticism at the table. Heated discussions trigger the sympathetic nervous system, which shuts down digestion.

There you go. Bring meaning to mealtime and enjoy benefits that go far beyond basic nourishment!

CHAPTER 5

Keto-Green Plant-Based Detox

Although you might be a confirmed omnivore like me (I eat everything except dairy), I recommend that you pause from animal foods at least two to three times a year (or more), in 6-day cycles. This is a beneficial tool for health and hormone balance—something we have learned from lots of studies.

Go on This Plan If You:

- Are a vegan or vegetarian.
- Want a break from animal products periodically, which I highly recommend.
- Have these symptoms of menopause: digestive problems (bloating, constipation, irritable bowel syndrome, and so forth), sleep disturbances, hot flashes, night sweats, and weight gain.
- Need to lose weight steadily.
- Have been diagnosed with hormonal imbalances or abnormal blood lipids (high triglycerides and high total cholesterol), or you've been told you're at risk for heart disease.
- Want to explore the plant-based lifestyle.

I wrote about plant-based eating in my *Keto-Green 16* book, which features a vegan plan. Plant-based diets are very popular—and for good reason. This nutritional approach does the following for you:

Helps Your Heart

A landmark trial analyzed the dietary patterns of about 96,000 Seventh-Day Adventists in the United States and Canada. These people ate with a wide variety of styles: vegan, vegetarian, pesco-vegetarian, semi-vegetarian, and nonvegetarian. According to the analysis, the risk for heart disease—the number-one killer in women—was lower among vegans and vegetarians. The reason for this was that vegans and vegetarians consume more fiber and have diets that are richer in alkalinizers and antioxidants.

Fiber is a nutritional miracle worker. We need it more now than ever before. It helps balance blood sugar and it produces satiety after meals. It keeps us regular and prevents constipation. It creates a healthy microbiome that is well populated

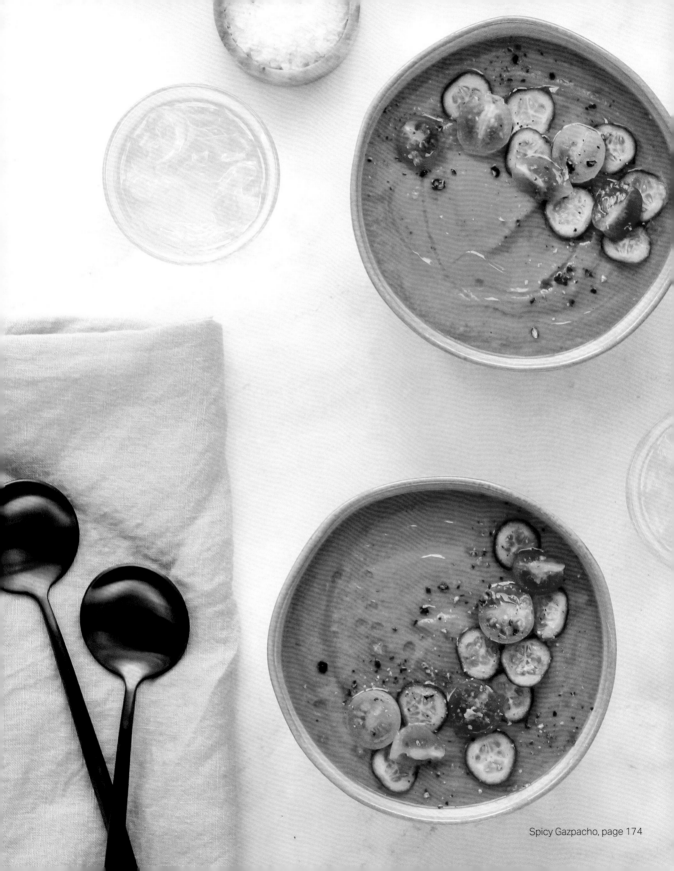

Spicy Gazpacho, page 174

with friendly gut bacteria, which in turn supports weight control, immunity, and hormone balance. In fact, studies suggest that if you eat more fiber, you'll keep your estrogen levels from fluctuating wildly.

As for antioxidants, they fight disease-causing free radicals. These free radicals are unstable atoms or molecules that contain one or more unpaired electrons in their outer orbit. Because of this, the free radicals attempt to become stable by "stealing" electrons from cell membranes.

Like the borders of your garden that keep weeds from invading your planting area, cell membranes protect the cells from free-radical invasion. If the cell membranes are penetrated by these molecular invaders, more free radicals—like fast-growing weeds—are generated. A chain reaction is set into motion that eventually results in inflammation, cellular damage, and disease. In the short term, free-radical attacks can make you feel inflamed and foggy-brained; in the longer term, they can cause memory loss, heart disease, stroke, Parkinson's disease, and many degenerative diseases. The more plant foods you eat and the more antioxidants you take in to promote your health, the more you will ease menopause issues and create a healthy microbiome with a diversity of beneficial gut bacteria.

Yields Quick Results

It doesn't take long to reap these benefits of a plant-based diet. One study showed that a dietary reset to plant-based eating can regenerate your health in a relatively short amount of time. In one study, researchers looked at 75 people—men and women—who were members of the Ethiopian Orthodox Christian Church. Their practice is to pause from animal foods around Lent. They follow a purely plant-based diet that involves eating whole grains, cereals, green leafy vegetables, legumes, peas, beans, and fruits.

The researchers assessed the subjects prior to starting the fast from animal foods, during Lent (seven weeks), and 7 weeks after the end of the Lenten (week 14). The results of this study were dramatic: the participants experienced significantly lower blood pressure, lower weight, and lower cholesterol levels after those seven weeks. The findings were even more pronounced in women than in men.

Balances Your Hormones

Plant-based nutrition has been associated with more balanced hormones. Foods such as beans, peas, and lentils are rich in natural estrogen and help balance that hormone within your body. Green leafy vegetables, including kale, spinach, and Swiss chard, can also help you maintain hormonal balance.

Science stands behind all this. In a survey of 754 premenopausal and postmenopausal women who were either vegans or omnivores, the vegans reported fewer hot flashes, night sweats, heart palpitations, changes in blood pressure, and other bothersome physical symptoms than did the omnivores.

Consider this, too. *U.S. News & World Report* recently reported that menopausal women who lose weight in the context of a healthy plant-based diet (meaning a diet rich in fruits, vegetables, legumes, nuts, and whole grains) can greatly reduce or eliminate their hot flashes and night sweats.

You'll be enjoying lots of cruciferous vegetables, such as broccoli, cabbage, cauliflower, bok choy, and Brussels sprouts on this plan—all of which contain high amounts of glucosinolates. These are natural detoxifying substances that help usher harmful estrogens from the body.

Offers Other Life-Saving Advantages

As for other benefits of a plant-based diet, we know from available evidence that plant-based eating can help you:

- Maintain a healthy weight
- Reduce your cancer risk
- Prevent Type 2 diabetes
- Boost your immune system
- Decrease inflammation
- Improve your digestive health
- Increase alkalinity
- Boost your mineral intake
- Ease joint pain
- Supercharge detoxification
- Strengthen your bones
- Improve your sleep quality
- Enjoy more energy
- Support longevity

So, if you're someone who would like to try plant-based eating or already a confirmed plant-based eater, this is definitely the right course of action.

What to Eat

A plant-based diet offers lots of variety, probably more than many other plans:

Vegetables: Pretty much any and all fresh, low-carbohydrate, high-fiber vegetables are on the table, like leafy greens, lettuce, tomatoes, spinach, broccoli, bok choy, mushrooms, Brussels sprouts, cauliflower, cucumbers, peppers, summer squash, and zucchini.

Protein: My favorite plant-based protein sources are beans, tempeh, tofu, lentils, and chickpeas. Green peas and edamame are also great options. Choose non-GMO sources whenever possible.

Nuts and Seeds: Almonds, cashews, walnuts, chia seeds, flax seeds, and hemp seeds are all staples in this kitchen. Nut butters and nut milks, too! All these foods contain protein and healthy fats.

Chia seeds and flax seeds also make great substitutes for eggs in baking—just one more reason to give them a try.

Healthy Fats: Extra-virgin olive oil, coconut oil, MCT oil, avocado oil, walnut oil, and olives are important to have on hand.

Herbs and Spices: Don't forget these; they're loaded with antioxidants and hormone-balancing phytonutrients. My favorites are garlic (technically a vegetable), oregano, basil, thyme, mint, sage, rosemary, cinnamon, nutmeg, and cardamom.

The bottom line here is that eating a plant-based diet is definitely helpful for women in the tenacious stages of hormone shifts, as well as for women who don't like animal products or don't want to eat them all the time and prefer a natural plant-based diet to manage their symptoms.

The Keto-Green Plant-Based Detox 6-Day Plan

Note: Each recipe makes two servings, with the exceptions of shakes and smoothies (which make 1 serving). So, feel free to have leftovers for any meal.

For a downloadable menu plan with a graphic representation of the meals, go to dranna.com/menupause-extras.

Day 1

Breakfast
Grain-Free Granola, with 6 ounces (¾ cup) nut milk or coconut milk yogurt

Lunch
Tahini Cauliflower Soup AND Mexican Mushrooms

Dinner
Miso-Ginger Zoodle Ramen

Day 2

Breakfast
Dr. Anna's Basic Keto-Green Meal Replacement Shake (see page 120)

Lunch
Spicy Gazpacho

Dinner
Kale and Tempeh Tacos

Day 3

Breakfast
Leftover Grain-Free Granola, with 6 ounces (¾ cup) nut milk or coconut milk yogurt

Lunch
Arabic Garden Salad and Dr. Anna's Keto-Green Tabbouleh

Dinner
Mushroom and Kale Stew AND Tomato Salad

Day 4

Breakfast
Garden Salad in a Shake

Lunch
Red Lentil and Squash Soup

Dinner
Comforting Spinach and Chickpeas

Day 5

Breakfast
Leftover Grain-Free Granola with 6 ounces
(¾ cup) nut milk or coconut milk yogurt

Lunch
Leftover Red Lentil and Squash Soup OR
Keto-Green Hummus WITH Jicama Salad

Dinner
Stovetop Ratatouille

Day 6

Breakfast
Garden Salad in a Shake

Lunch
Golden Cabbage Chickpea Soup

Dinner
Roasted Cauliflower Steaks WITH Tangle
of Greens

You Can DIY Your Meals

Although I recommend that you follow the 6-day plan as outlined, feel free to create your own meals for breakfast, lunch, and dinner. Simply DIY your meals by following this template:

Breakfast: + 1 plant-based protein serving + 1 serving of vegetables + 1 serving of fat.

An example might be a smoothie made with 1 cup coconut milk, a scoop of recommended protein powder, a handful of spinach, and 1 tablespoon of almond butter.

Lunch: 1 plant-based protein serving + 1 to 2 servings vegetables + 1 to 2 fat servings.

An example might be ½ to 1 cup black soybeans; 1 to 2 cups spinach, kale, or beet greens sautéed in 1 tablespoon olive oil or coconut oil or avocado oil; and ½ avocado, sliced.

Dinner = 1 plant-based protein serving + 2 servings vegetables + 1 to 2 fat servings.

An example might be 1 cup kidney beans, cauliflower rice, and a side salad with fresh greens and 1 tablespoon hemp seeds, tossed with 1 tablespoon olive oil and the juice of ½ or 1 lemon.

Your 6-Day Shopping List

You may not need to purchase all these items; you probably have many of them in your kitchen or pantry right now. Also, what you buy depends on which menu options you choose, or whether you DIY some of your meals. This shopping list is based on using all the recipes in the menus. It is designed for two people, so if you are cooking for yourself, purchase only half of each item, depending on how it is sold.

For a downloadable shopping list, go to dranna.com/menupause-extras.

Supplements and Staples to Have On Hand

Dr. Anna's Keto-Green or Keto-Alkaline mix; or a good substitute protein powder, formulated with a vegan protein such as pea or rice protein and containing less than 3 grams of sugar (per serving) and less than 10 grams of carbohydrate (per serving)

Mighty Maca Plus, 7.2-ounce container; or 1 (4-ounce) bag powdered maca root

Coconut oil, 1 (14-ounce) jar

Extra-virgin olive oil, 1 (16-ounce) bottle

Vegetable oil cooking spray, 1 (7-ounce) can

Sherry vinegar, 1 small bottle

White wine vinegar, 1 small bottle

Coconut aminos, 1 (16-ounce) bottle

Vanilla extract, small bottle

Tahini, 1 (16-ounce) jar

Seasonings: sea salt, black pepper, ground cinnamon, ground nutmeg, ground allspice, ground cumin, ground coriander, chili powder, paprika, turmeric powder, cayenne, minced preserved lemon, Za'atar blend (or dried thyme), red pepper flakes

Dried herbs: Mexican oregano, mint

Seeds and Nuts

Sunflower seeds, hulled, unsalted, 1 (3.5-ounce) bag

Pumpkin seeds, hulled, unsalted, 1 (3.5-ounce) bag

Hemp seeds, 1 (.5-ounce) bag

Sesame seeds, 1 (8-ounce) jar

Cumin seeds, 1 (2-ounce) jar

Coriander seeds, 1 (2-ounce) jar

Almonds, sliced, 1 (14-ounce) bag

Pecans, chopped, 1 (16-ounce) bag

Pine nuts, 1 (4-ounce) bag

Pili nuts, 1 (4-ounce) bag

Coconut flakes, unsweetened, 1 (7-ounce) bag

Produce—Fresh Vegetables

Spinach, 2 or 3 (16-ounce) bags (1 bag can be baby spinach)

Arugula, 5 ounces or 2½ cups

Romaine lettuce, 1 head

Lettuce, any type, 1 small head

Red lettuce, 1 small bunch

Kale, 1 (16-ounce) bag

Tuscan kale, 1 (16-ounce) bag

Mustard greens, 1 (16-ounce) bag

Green cabbage, 2 small heads

Radishes, 1 small bunch

Cucumbers, 3 medium, 1 large

Carrots, 2 medium

Celery, 2 stalks

Yellow onions, 2 small, 6 medium, 1 large

Red onion, 1 small
Shallots, 3
Scallions, 1 bunch
Garlic, 4 to 5 bulbs
Green bell pepper, 2
Fresh ginger, 1 (4-inch) piece
White button mushrooms, 1 (16-ounce) package
Shiitake mushrooms, 2 (16-ounce) packages
Wild mushrooms, 1 (4-ounce) package
Tomatoes, Roma (plum), 1 pound
Tomatoes, slicing, 6 medium
Cherry tomatoes, 1 pint
Zucchini, 2 medium, 1 large
Eggplant, 1 medium
Jicama, 1 small
Butternut squash, 1 medium
Cauliflower, 1 small head, 1 large head
Broccoli sprouts, 1 (4 ounce) container
Red bell pepper, 1

Produce—Fresh Herbs
Cilantro, 1 bunch
Mint, 1 (.5-ounce) package or 1 bunch
Parsley, 2 bunches
Thyme, 1 (.5-ounce) package or 1 bunch

Produce—Fresh Fruits
Avocados, medium
Lemons, 9
Limes, 3
Oranges, 3

Legumes and Plant Proteins
Red lentils, 1 (16-ounce) package
Chickpeas, 3 (14-ounce) cans
White miso paste, 1 (16-ounce) container
Tempeh, 1 (4-ounce) package

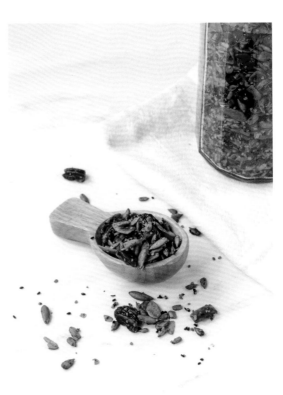

Non-Dairy Milks and Milk Products
Unsweetened coconut milk, 1 quart
Full-fat coconut milk, 1 (14-ounce) can
Unsweetened coconut yogurt, 3 (6-ounce) containers

Other Items
Tomatoes, diced, 1 (28-ounce) can
Vegetable broth, 5 (32-ounce) packages
Minced garlic, 1 (4.5-ounce) jar
Strawberries, frozen, 1 (10-ounce) bag
Dried cherries, 1 (5-ounce) package

Strategies for Success

1. Follow this plan exactly as written or substitute any meal with DIY meals you create based on the food lists.

2. You have the option of intermittent fasting on this plan. This type of fasting condenses your entire food intake to a specific window of time. A popular way to begin this is to have 16 hours of fasting and 8 hours of feeding, or a ratio of 16:8. So, for example, if you have your last meal at 6:00 p.m., you wouldn't eat the next day until after 10:00 a.m. And, yes, sleeping time counts toward fasting! Intermittent fasting helps with weight loss, reduced inflammation, cellular renewal, detoxification, and other conditions.

   Alternatively, you may feel that you require only two meals daily in an 8-hour eating window, and having just two meals feels satisfying. This is an effective way to eat, because it encourages weight loss.

3. Test your urinary pH and ketones first thing in the morning (and periodically throughout the day whenever you go to the bathroom), with the goal of keeping your pH at or above 7.0. The pinker the strip, the higher your level of ketosis (fat-burning). Record everything in a journal. (See dranna.com/menupause-extras for a downloadable journal page and how to order my test strips.)

4. Weigh yourself each morning so as to monitor your weight loss.

5. Hydrate! Drink approximately half your ideal body weight in ounces of filtered water each day. But don't drink more than 4 ounces (½ cup) of fluids with any given meal, so that your digestive juices have time to do their work. My typical recommendation is to drink water up to 20 minutes before you eat, then have 4 ounces (½ cup) of fluid with your meal, and wait one to two hours afterward.

6. Never overload your stomach. When you begin to feel full, stop eating. And remember, do not snack.

7. Do not eat between meals and do not snack. Snacking can be destructive to your goals. It can cause insulin resistance, weight gain, hot flashes, and inflammation. If you feel hunger pangs during the day, see the snacking options discussed earlier. You can add more healthy fats and oils to green leafy salads, or enjoy a large cup of Dr. Anna's Mineral Broth (page 244).

8. If you enjoy plant-based eating, and are making progress on it, continue the plan for further 6-day cycles until you reach your happy weight—or longer. If it is working for you, stay with it. Or, feel free to try any of the other plans in this book. Record how you feel on each plan and note the progress you are making. (See dranna.com/menupause-extras for a downloadable journal page.)

Menopause Around the World: The Seventh-Day Adventists of Loma Linda

For a look at what a plant-based lifestyle can do for you in your menopausal years and beyond, look no further than the Seventh-Day Adventist women living in Loma Linda, California. Most of them follow a vegetarian regimen that encourages a well-balanced diet, including nuts, fruits, and legumes, and one that is low in sugar, salt, and refined grains. According to research, women who follow this kind of diet have better glucose control, lower total cholesterol levels, and lower LDL cholesterol than nonvegetarians, meaning their risk of heart disease is much lower. In fact, recent research has found that people who live this lifestyle have the nation's lowest rates of heart disease and diabetes and very low rates of overweight or obesity.

Also, the diets of these women are much higher in vitamins and minerals than those of nonvegetarians, which means they're getting all the immune-boosting benefits these nutrients provide.

Their plant-based diet appears to be cancer protective, too. These women who ate tomatoes three or four times a week slashed their chance of getting ovarian cancer by 70 percent, compared with those who ate tomatoes less often. What's more, these women experienced lower mortality rates from breast cancer than did other white females in the United States. Other studies have shown that Seventh-Day Adventists who ate legumes such as peas and beans three times a week had a 30 to 40 percent reduction in colon cancer.

Pretty amazing, right? If you've never considered going vegan or vegetarian, the next 6 days can be a great introduction to it. Be sure to try as many of the *MenuPause* plant-based recipes as you can.

CHAPTER 6

The Carbohydrate Pause

Picture this: for breakfast, you dig into some crispy bacon and yummy eggs. When lunchtime hits, you enjoy delicate, bite-sized pieces of sashimi, dipped in a little wasabi. For dinner, you grill a few juicy beef burgers—hold the cheese. And the buns. And the veggies. Or, how about steak and lobster at a fine restaurant?

You're living the meat-lover's dream. It's known as the "zero-carb diet," or as I've designed it, the Carbohydrate Pause. The principles of this plan are simple: you temporarily eat only animal foods while pausing all carbs. There is no counting of calories or macros or measuring of portions. You eat when you're hungry and stop when you're full. That's it.

Carb-pausing is a great way to smash through a weight-loss plateau, rapidly get the scale moving in a lower direction, and claim many other health benefits that are important concerning menopause.

Go on This Plan If You:

- Want to stimulate rapid weight loss
- Want to smash a plateau
- Are "weight-loss resistant," meaning you have trouble dropping pounds
- Have an autoimmune disease
- Are insulin resistant
- Have menopause symptoms such as insulin resistance, sudden weight gain, hard-to-budge belly fat, cravings, sleep disturbances, frequent bloating, and brain fog

We humans actually evolved as meat-eaters, surviving on meats, wild turkey, and the fats within them, especially during winter. Our ancestors ate very few plant foods. And this is why we have incisor teeth for biting and molars for grinding.

Following a no-carbohydrate diet is a great reset that takes the body back to its nutritional roots. Further, meat is a nutrient-dense food, loaded with vitamins, minerals, essential amino acids, and other health-building nutrients. In fact, there are several nutrients we require for good health that can only be found in animal foods, such as meat, poultry, and seafood. True, this plan, as well as meat-eating in general, is not for everyone, and I respect that. But if you do enjoy meat and need a change or a jump-start for weight loss, the Carbohydrate Pause is worth a try.

Opposite: Spicy Diablo Eggs, page 196

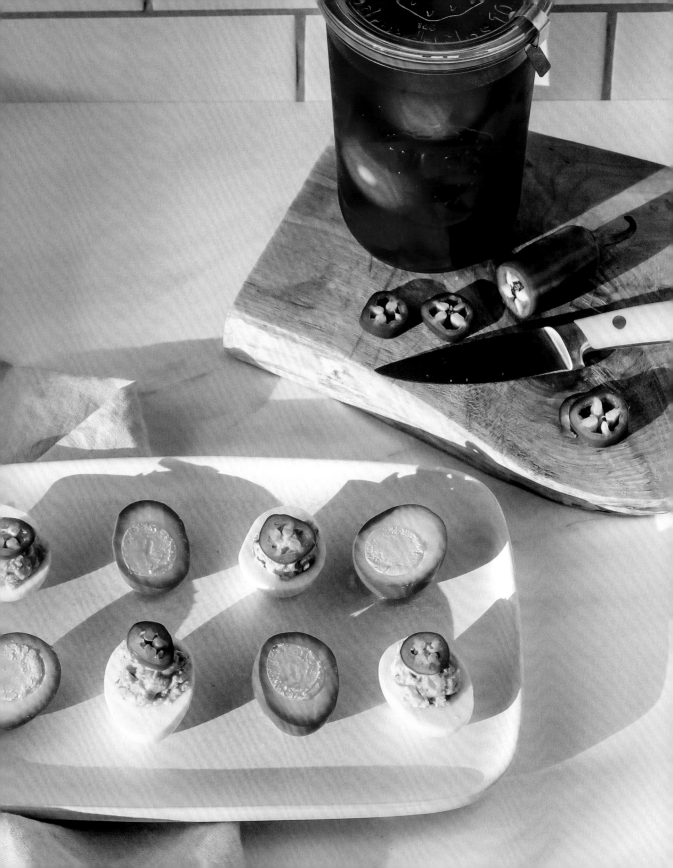

Probing the Power of Protein

What can you expect while following this plan? Although not everyone will want to try this, research indicates that it offers some impressive benefits, as follows:

Rapid Weight Loss

This plan is obviously high in protein, which has numerous weight-loss benefits. First, since an all-meat and seafood diet will put you into ketosis rather quickly, you can expect to lose a pound a day or more while pausing carbs. Protein is also highly filling (*satiating* is the technical word), a factor that leads to reduced caloric intake and subsequent weight loss. Protein also increases your metabolic rate, helping you burn more calories.

Loss of muscle mass can occur during menopause. Because "muscle is metabolism," a loss means your body can't burn fat as well. The solution is to up your protein intake.

Therefore, following the Carbohydrate Pause will likely cause you to feel fuller and lighter overall.

Hormone Balance

Meat and seafood have a big say in how your hormones work. Primarily, they are useful in boosting testosterone levels. This means that this plan can be effective in relieving estrogen dominance, a cause of weight gain and other problems during menopause. Menopausal women need testosterone for other reasons, which are to preserve and increase libido, retain muscle mass, and avoid disorders like osteoporosis and depression.

The reason meat raises testosterone is that it contains lots of zinc, which promotes testosterone production in the body.

Eating fish, in particular, is a great way to raise progesterone levels, because it is high in vitamin D, a nutrient that promotes progesterone production. Progesterone is very important for brain health, anti-anxiety, and improved sleep, among other benefits.

Anti-Aging

You have different nutritional needs when you reach menopause; your body is different (and in lots of ways better!) than it was at age 25. One of your most pressing needs right now is more protein. Protein is the youth macronutrient, especially for women! Here's why:

Protein helps you stay healthy into your later years. In one study of more than 300 elderly participants (average age of 72), women who consumed between 1.75 to 2.65 grams of protein per pound of body weight each day tended to have fewer health problems than women eating less than 1.75 grams. So, if you weigh 150 pounds, you'll want to eat at least 260 grams of protein daily.

Protein makes you strong and functional. In your 30s, your muscle mass begins to gradually fall off; after age 50, this decline speeds up. However, if you eat enough protein and engage in regular resistance training, you can put a stop to this decline and actually increase your lean muscle mass and strength.

Protein gives you the power of amino acids. Amino acids are the building blocks of protein, which in turn make up the structure of our body's cells, muscles, and tissues. Although they are not as popular or as widely known as vitamins and minerals, they play a significant role in menopausal health. There are many different kinds of amino acids, but a few of them are specifically beneficial for women who are in the menopausal stage.

One is arginine, found in meat, especially poultry and pork, seeds like pumpkin seeds, and legumes such as peanuts, chickpeas, and lentils. A good supply of arginine supports blood vessel elasticity and reduces the frequency of hot flashes.

Another is lysine, widely available in beef, chicken, pork, tuna, king crab, and firm tofu. Lysine has lots of menopausal benefits. It helps your body better absorb calcium, thus helping prevent osteoporosis. It works together with arginine to support the integrity of your blood vessels and further reduce hot flashes. And it controls the buildup of too many lipids in your arteries, helping prevent heart disease—the number-one killer of women.

Then we have the branched-chain amino acids, valine, leucine, and isoleucine (BCAAs). Prevalent in animal proteins, the BCAAs ensure that your body is always making muscle. Of the three, leucine is the standout. Its number-one job is to enhance muscle growth by stimulating the body to manufacture muscle. Leucine has also been found to trigger fat-burning.

If you limit your consumption of animal protein, you risk not having enough BCAAs to ensure that muscle protein synthesis outweighs muscle protein breakdown.

Another amino acid that is important in anti-aging is carnitine, found in meat. Technically, it is considered "conditionally essential," yet I feel it is essential and I recommend carnitine supplements to obtain even more.

Carnitine has so many benefits. It has been praised as a nutrient to help fight Alzheimer's disease and as an anti-aging supplement because it improves memory function. By far, the most important anti-aging effect carnitine has, however, is to maintain the function of the mitochondria, the energy factories of our cells, especially heart cells. When mitochondrial function dwindles, degenerative disease and heart muscle weakness become inevitable consequences. Carnitine has been shown to reverse heart aging.

Strengthens Bones

A short supply of protein not only contributes to loss of muscle mass as you age but also affects bone loss. But when you consistently eat ample protein, expect greater bone density and bone strength.

A 2019 study conducted in the Netherlands analyzed four major studies, looking at high versus low protein

Collagen: The Super Anti-Aging Protein

I periodically cook up big batches of bone broth and sip cupfuls of it throughout the day. After a week or so of supplementing with bone broth like this, I notice that my skin, especially on my face, is glowing, firm, and youthful. These amazing changes are not the result of some expensive skincare product. They are a result of the collagen in the bone broth.

Yes, collagen! Collagen is a protein found naturally in the body that gives skin its firmness, elasticity, and youthful look. Some 25 to 35 percent of the protein in our body is collagen. Over time, that percentage decreases due to age-related hormonal changes, sun exposure, environmental insults, and stress. As we approach our 40s, we lose about a teaspoon of collagen a year. The result is loose skin, sagging under the chin, and wrinkles—all of which can worsen over time.

Bone broth has other healing benefits beyond skin. It is a major healer of our bones and joints. In fact, there are more than 60 scientific studies proving the effectiveness of collagen for improving joint pain, osteoarthritis, bone-density loss (osteoporosis), and skin aging.

Fortunately, you can boost your body's own collagen production to achieve a fresher, tighter, more youthful complexion in three important ways.

First, you can try drinking bone broth the way I do. You can buy it in most grocery stores these days, but I love my own brews. Simply boil any animal bones—beef, bison, chicken, turkey, fish (ideally bones from organic sources)—for 16 to 24 hours in order to release all the goodness. Throw in some veggies like greens, onions, and garlic, too. (See my recipes on pages 240–246.)

Here's a tip: You can tell whether your broth has a lot of collagen in it after you refrigerate it: if it gels in the fridge, it's full of collagen.

The second way is to supplement with collagen powder. This type of supplement is trendy right now, but there is good science behind it as well. Research has shown that you can increase your body's collagen levels by consuming more collagen through supplementation, no matter what your age. It is available in powders you can mix into coffee, tea, smoothies, and other beverages. These collagen supplements can renew and revitalize the way you look and feel (it's good for joints, too). Collagen's benefits were confirmed in a 2019 article published in the *Journal of Drugs in Dermatology*. After looking into eight different studies, the researchers concluded: "Oral collagen supplements also increase skin elasticity, hydration, and dermal collagen density. Collagen supplementation is generally safe with no reported adverse events."

The third way to pump up your collagen intake is to stir collagen powder into your bone broth. You get a nice double dose of this remarkable anti-aging protein that way.

Check out the Resources section of this book, and visit drannacabeca.com/menupause-extras for my favorite collagen products.

consumption and bone health in people over age 65. The investigators found that higher protein intakes resulted in a significant decrease in hip fractures.

This is an important and promising finding, because hip fractures are a major cause of death and disability. In a review of studies published between 1957 and 2009 (involving a total of 578,436 women and 154,276 men over the age of 50), researchers noted that the risk of death in both men and women in the three months after a hip fracture was between five and eight times higher.

So—take protein seriously. At the same time, please follow the portion recommendations for protein. Like anything else, you can eat too much protein. Excessive protein can turn into glucose in the body, creating weight-loss resistance, inflammation, and weight gain.

Brainpower

When you start forgetting things mid-sentence, feeling fuzzy in the head, or losing focus, it can feel as if you're going crazy. And it's scary. I understand because I've been there. There was a time I was so overwhelmed by all that was happening in my life that it led to a serious case of brain fog.

Fortunately, this assault on our thinking, our concentration, our hormonal balance, and even how we adapt to stress can be overturned with food, particularly protein.

You have probably seen plenty of headlines about the omega-3 fatty acids in fish. These nutrients positively influence the course of so many conditions and illnesses. In terms of brain health, omega-3 fats are beneficial in promoting better clarity, mood, and overall thinking. What's more, they also help improve concentration and the general operation of your brain—good news if you frequently experience brain fog.

Another nutrient in animal protein that helps brain fog is choline, a neurotransmitter that is involved in sleep, muscle control, pain regulation, learning, and memory. Choline is available only from animal foods, most notably eggs and liver.

Vitamin B_{12} is another brain-protective nutrient. A deficiency of vitamin B_{12} has been suggested as a culprit for depressed cognitive function in people who consume only vegetable foods. Guess where you can get B_{12}? Animal protein!

Animal proteins, in particularly beef, are also rich in carnitine. Many human studies show that carnitine improves mental function and reduces deterioration in older adults with mild cognitive impairment and Alzheimer's disease.

So, yes, a meat-rich diet might just bring your brain out of the fog and into the clear.

Improves Hair and Skin

All my life, I've been incredibly proud of my long, thick hair. Then it happened: dark hairs on my pillow. My shower drain plugged with clumps of hair. My hair falling out in handfuls. The shine and volume were gone. This added to my depression. Was I going bald?

And I am not alone. I've had many patients bring their hair in plastic bags. Feeling very stressed, they had pulled their hair from shower drains and off pillows, too, to prove their hair loss. I know how distressful this is.

What was the reason for the demise of our crowning glory? In my case, early menopause brought on by premature ovarian failure and extreme stress and PTSD. In my patients' cases, the reasons were similar—hormonal changes brought on by menopause, stress, and in many instances, insufficient protein in their diets.

It has been estimated that by the time we reach the age of 60, roughly 80 percent of women worldwide will be dealing with some degree of hair loss. If this is happening to you, you are not alone, and there are solutions. For starters, look no further than what you put on your plate.

There is a lot of impressive research concerning omega-3 fatty acids when it comes to hair growth. One of the many studies that really intrigued me was published in 2015 in the *Journal of Cosmetic Dermatology*. It clearly shows that supplementing with omega-3 fatty acids, plus omega-6s and antioxidants, not only regrew hair in women but also thickened it.

For healing your skin, there's more good news about omega-3 fatty acids specifically. In a 2010 report in *Clinics in Dermatology*, the researchers wrote: "These fatty acids are showing promise as safe adjunctive treatments for many skin disorders, including atopic dermatitis,

psoriasis, acne vulgaris, systemic lupus erythematosus, nonmelanoma skin cancer, and melanoma."

Check out the Resources section of this book and visit dranna.com/menupause-extras for my recommended omega-3 fatty acid supplement.

Cardiovascular Health

My family history is significant in regard to heart disease. In fact, my mother struggled for years with it, and when she was only 52 (and I was 16) she underwent cardiac bypass surgery. That crisis spurred me to become a vegetarian; in the 1980s, we were led to believe that heavy meat consumption was a cause of heart disease. I stayed a vegetarian for 12 years. But I struggled with my weight and anemia the entire time, and finally, while in med school, realized I needed more protein. My diet was too carb heavy and protein and fat poor. One day, after practicing my suturing on raw chicken thighs, I ended up stuffing, seasoning, and cooking them—delicious!

Now we know that meat is not bad for your heart, as some sources suggested. It can be part of a heart-healthy diet— for several reasons. First, both meat and fish contain those wonderful omega-3 fats, which help cut the risk of irregular heartbeats, stroke, and heart attack.

Meat is also packed with iron. As we know, iron is one of the most important minerals in ensuring the transport of oxygen to the cells and proper blood circulation.

Although meat does contain cholesterol (as do all animal products), the government's latest dietary recommendations have removed the limit on cholesterol consumption. This is because studies now suggest that dietary cholesterol has very little effect on blood cholesterol.

What's more, studies now show that low-carbohydrate diets (such as this one) are equally effective as low-fat diets in reducing weight and improving cardiovascular risk factors. Thus, there's some definite value in a high-meat diet with regard to heart health.

Strengthens Immunity

Because meat has such an excellent nutrient profile, it is beneficial in boosting your immune system. The key immunity players in meat are:

Omega-3 fatty acids. These wonder-working fats help the body fight harmful infections.

Vitamin B6. This vitamin is involved in regulating the production of infection-fighting white blood cells. Beef, in particular, contains more than twice the amount of vitamin B6 as soybeans, lentils, and other vegetable protein sources. A short supply of this vitamin can decrease the production of certain immune-system cells.

Protein. This nutrient is a vital immune booster, responsible for manufacturing protective antibodies. A protein-deficient diet can impair wound and fracture healing and reduce your ability to fight infection. In general, animal proteins are superior to vegetable proteins in keeping your immune system strong.

Zinc. For strong immunity, zinc is essential. It is a veritable Fort Knox when it comes to protecting against infection and disease. The most shining example surfaced during the Covid-19 outbreak in 2020, when scientists at Sechenov University in Moscow published the news in a remarkable review that zinc could protect against Covid-19 by supporting antiviral immunity and reducing inflammation.

Above-average dietary sources of zinc include oysters (my favorite), liver (so good for you that I forced myself to eat it recently and enjoyed it), and free-range and grass-fed meat (see page 79). See my recipe for Super Burgers (page 202) to get a lot of this nutritional goodness.

Fights Inflammation

Generally, plant foods are among the most powerful of all inflammation fighters. But there is also an amino acid in animal proteins that reduces inflammation: taurine. It increases the action of antioxidants to protect cell tissue from damage. At the same time, it inhibits the creation of pro-inflammatory agents and free radicals that cause inflammation.

Animal products are quite rich in taurine, whereas plant products are devoid of this amino acid. For this reason, if you don't eat animal products, you are likely to have poor taurine status. But again, stick to the recommended portions of protein. In excess, protein can trigger inflammation.

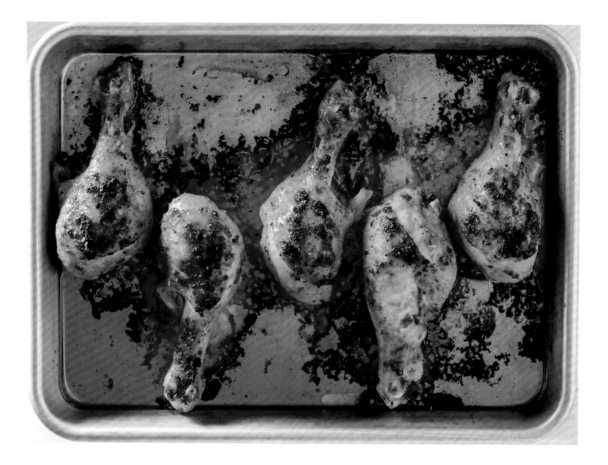

Helps with Autoimmune Conditions

All-meat diets got in the spotlight based on rumors that they reduce symptoms of autoimmune disease—conditions in which your immune system mistakenly attacks your body (like asthma, celiac disease, Hashimoto's, lupus, and rheumatoid arthritis). The theory is that a zero-carb diet eliminates foods and ingredients that may cause the body to turn against itself.

While there are not yet many studies looking into the autoimmune effect of this diet, there are many anecdotal reports and testimonials about how diets high in animal products are relieving people of autoimmune conditions and the inflammation associated with it.

Above: Easy Roasted Drumsticks, page 227

Which Animal Proteins Are the Best?

The Carbohydrate Pause consists mostly of meat and animal products. Foods to eat include beef, bison, chicken, pork, lamb, turkey, organ meats, fish, and shellfish. You don't have to count calories or measure serving sizes; simply eat until you feel satisfied.

Non-Processed Meats

For optimal health, it is best to buy foods containing the fewest ingredients possible. They are generally less processed, with fewer toxins, because they are closer to their original form. Most meats fit this category. They don't have an ingredient list because the food itself is the only ingredient (the same applies to fresh and frozen vegetables). An exception here is processed meats such as hot dogs, bologna, and various luncheon meats. They come with a fairly lengthy list of additives and should be avoided.

Grass-Fed Meat

You are what you eat, but you are also what your food eats (or gets injected). Put another way, when you eat meats from healthy animals, you become healthier yourself. So, you want to purchase grass-fed meat for the best nutritional outcomes. Grass-fed cattle have higher levels of omega-3 fats than grain-fed cattle, and they have fewer bacterial infections and parasites (meaning they require fewer antibiotics).

Organically Raised Poultry

There are three important reasons to look for poultry and eggs that are organically raised and pasture-raised ("USDA Organic"). First, organic-poultry growers are legally prohibited from using sewage sludge as fertilizer, most synthetic chemicals, or genetically modified organisms (GMOs), which would be any plant, animal, or microorganism that has been altered through genetic engineering.

Second, pasture-raised birds are healthier. If the birds are crowded together in cages, which is what conventional growers do, they're more likely to produce infectious bacteria. They are then fed antibiotics, traces of which ultimately get into our bodies. USDA Organic chickens, on the other hand, are allowed access to the outdoors and rarely require antibiotics.

Third, eating organic chicken may prevent you from getting food poisoning. In a 2010 study, fewer than 6 percent of organic birds were infected with salmonella, compared with almost 39 percent of conventional ones.

Wild-Caught Seafood

Wild-caught seafood is fish that has been caught in a natural habitat (lake, ocean, river), whereas farmed seafood is raised in large tanks or pools. Check the labels to ensure that your seafood is indeed wild-caught.

As with other animals, the nutritional quality of the seafood largely depends on what the fish eats. Fish in the wild eat a natural diet and tend to be free of the diseases and contaminants commonly found in farm-raised fish.

You've probably heard a lot about mercury levels in fish. It is wise to be cautious here, because mercury is a dangerous brain and nervous-system toxin. The highest levels of mercury in fish are found in the large predatory species. These include shark, swordfish, king mackerel, and tilefish. Other types of fish, as well as shellfish, have less mercury and are safer to eat.

Does the quality of seafood differ depending on where it is sourced? In short, yes. Imported seafood is not guaranteed to be as regulated as domestic. For one thing, imported farm-raised fish tends to be high in antibiotics. What's more, many international fish farms are not held to the same high inspection standards that are imposed in the United States. To check the origins, you can look at the Country of Origin Labeling (COOL), which is required on all seafood sold in the United States.

Eggs

People often categorize eggs as dairy, but eggs are the "fruit" of chickens, whereas dairy comes from cows (and a few other animals). Eggs contain no dairy products such as whey, casein, and lactose, while offering the highest biological value of any protein. Eggs are also packed with vitamin A, various B vitamins, minerals, and phytonutrients. For the healthiest selection, look for cage-free eggs.

The bottom line is that we must do everything possible to eliminate the toxins from our foods. Choosing organic, grass-fed, free-range, cage-free, and wild-caught foods is a vital step toward that goal.

The 6-Day Carbohydrate Pause

For a downloadable menu plan with a graphic representation of the meals, go to dranna.com/menupause-extras.

Day 1

Breakfast
Spicy Diablo Eggs

Lunch
Keto Texas Chili

Dinner
Creamy Coconut-Saffron Mussels OR Bacon-Wrapped Scallops

Day 2

Breakfast
Pickled Beet Eggs

Lunch
Leftover Keto Texas Chili OR Super Burgers (page 202)

Dinner
Southwestern Spiced Pork Tenderloin OR Ghee-Basted Pork Chops

Day 3

Breakfast
Crispy Keto Hash

Lunch
Bacon-Wrapped Chicken Tenders OR
Easy Roasted Drumsticks

Dinner
Kafta Kabobs OR
Beef Ribs with Bacon

Day 4

Breakfast
Scotch Eggs

Lunch
Classic Roast Chicken OR
Crispy Chicken Thighs

Dinner
Balsamic-Oregano Beef Heart OR
Ribeye Steak with Spiced Ghee

Day 5

Breakfast
Leftover Crispy Keto Hash

Lunch
Ginger-Soy Shredded Beef

Dinner
Garlic and Herbed Leg of Lamb

Day 6

Breakfast
Spicy Diablo Eggs

Lunch
Leftover Ginger-Soy Shredded Beef

Dinner
Crispy Skin Salmon OR
Vinegar-Poached Herby Fish

Your 6-Day Shopping List

For a downloadable shopping list of this plan, go to dranna.com/menupause-extras.

Staples to Have On Hand
Coconut oil, 1 (17-ounce) jar
Extra-virgin olive oil, 1 (16-ounce) bottle
Toasted sesame oil, 1 (5-ounce) bottle
Ghee (clarified butter), 1 (13-ounce) jar
Coconut aminos,* 1 (16-ounce) bottle
Distilled white vinegar, 1 (16-ounce) bottle
Apple cider vinegar, 1 quart
Balsamic vinegar (sugar-free), 1 (16-ounce) bottle
White wine vinegar, 1 small bottle
Minced garlic, 1 (4-ounce) jar
Ginger root, 2-inch piece
Sesame seeds
Ranch seasoning powder
Seasonings: sea salt, black pepper, white pepper, garlic powder, onion powder
Spices: ground allspice, ground cumin, chili powder, paprika, chipotle powder or smoked paprika, cayenne, saffron threads, habanero flakes
Dried herbs: oregano, thyme, bay leaves

*Note: This is a healthier choice than soy sauce because it has no gluten, GMOs, MSG, or high amounts of sodium.

Produce—Fresh Vegetables

Jalapeño peppers, 2
Yellow onions, 2 medium, 1 large
Shallots, 2
Garlic, 1 bulb
Tomato, 1 medium, ripe

Produce—Fresh Herbs

Parsley, 1 bunch
Oregano, 1 (.5-ounce) package
Thyme, 1 (.5-ounce) package
Mint, 1 (.5-ounce) package or 1 bunch
Rosemary, 1 (.5-ounce) package

Produce—Fresh Fruit

Avocados, 2 medium
Lemons, 4
Lime, 1

Protein Sources

Eggs, large, 1 dozen
Mussels, in shell, 1 pound
Sea scallops, 1 pound
Salmon, 2 (4- to 6-ounce) fillets, skin on
Cod, 2 (4- to 6-ounce) fillets (or other firm-fleshed white fish)
Chicken livers, 1 (8-ounce) package
Chicken, roasting, 1 whole (about 3½ pounds)
Chicken tenders, 8 (about 1 pound)
Chicken drumsticks, 1 pound
Chicken thighs, skin-on, bone-in, 1 pound
Beef chuck roast, boneless, 1½ pounds
Beef back ribs, 1 pound
Beef ribeye, bone-in, 2 (6-ounce) steaks
Beef heart, 1 (about 3 pounds)
Beef, ground (preferably grass-fed), 1½ pound
Beef or bison, ground (preferably grass-fed), 1 pound (or ground turkey)

Lamb, ½ leg, with bone (3 to 4 pounds)
Lamb, ground (preferably grass-fed), 1 pound (or ground beef)
Pork tenderloin, 2 pounds
Pork chops, thick-cut, bone-in, 2 (8 ounces total)
Pork sausage, ground, 8 ounces
Bacon, 1 (1-pound) and 1 (8-ounce) package

Non-Dairy Milk

Coconut milk, full-fat, 1 (14-ounce) can

Other Items

Tomato paste, 1 (6-ounce) can
Beets, 1 (14-ounce) can (or 1 bunch fresh beets)
Capers, 1 (3.5-ounce) jar
Beef broth or beef bone broth, 2 (14.5-ounce) cans
Chicken broth, 1 (8-ounce) container or bone broth, 1 (14.5-ounce) can

Strategies for Success

1. Follow this plan exactly as written. However, you can create your own DIY meals, as long as it is an animal-based meal.
2. You have the option of intermittent fasting on this plan. This type of fasting condenses your entire food intake to a specific window of time. A popular way to begin this is 16 hours of fasting and 8 hours of feeding, or 16:8. So, for example, if you have your last meal at 6:00 p.m., you wouldn't eat the next day until after 10:00 a.m. And, yes, sleep

Opposite: Crispy Chicken Thighs, page 209

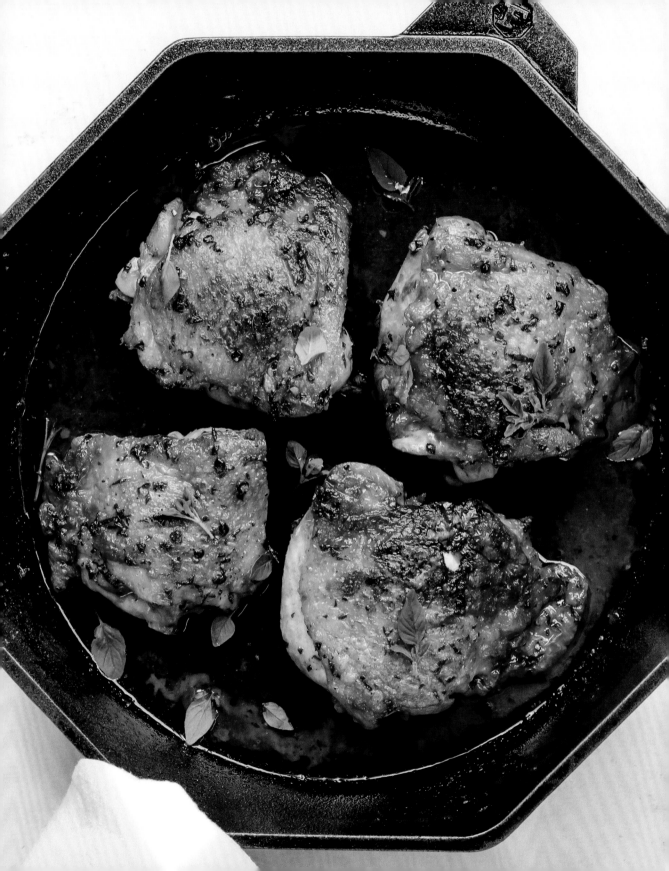

time counts toward fasting! Intermittent fasting helps with weight loss, reduced inflammation, cellular renewal, detoxification, and more.

Alternatively, you may feel that you require only two meals daily in an 8-hour eating window, and that having just two meals feels satisfying. This is an effective way to eat, because it encourages weight loss.

3. This plan will put you in ketosis, so use testing strips to test your ketones first thing in the morning (and periodically throughout the day or whenever you go to the bathroom). The pinker the strip, the higher your level of ketosis (fat-burning). For testing strips, go to the Resources section of this book or to dranna.com/menupause-extras. You'll find a wealth of tools to help you on this amazing journey.

4. Weigh yourself each morning to see how well you're losing weight.

5. Hydrate! An all-meat diet can be dehydrating so make sure you drink approximately half your ideal body weight in ounces of filtered water each day. But don't drink more than 4 ounces (½ cup) of fluids with any given meal, so that your digestive juices have time to do their work. My typical recommendation is to drink water up to 20 minutes before you eat, then have 4 ounces (½ cup) of fluid with your meal, and wait one to two hours afterward.

6. Never overload your stomach. When you begin to feel full, stop eating.

7. Do not eat between meals and do not snack. If you feel hungry, enjoy a large cup of one of my meat-based bone broths (see pages 240–246).

8. Take digestive enzyme supplements after each meal to help you digest all the protein. I suggest that you take 1 or 2 capsules after meals.

9. On day 6, observe how you have been feeling, particularly with regard to your symptoms. If you feel good and want to continue losing more weight, follow this plan for another 6 days. But do not stay on it for more than 12 days at a time, because it can be acidic to the body. A good transition is to switch to the 21-day Keto-Green Plan in *The Hormone Fix*. Doing so can maximize your results, and I've seen great outcomes when women do this. Carrie is a good example. She lost an additional 35 pounds after making this transition, and her lab results, including blood sugar, liver enzymes, and estrogen balance stabilized in normal ranges.

Menopause Around the World: Inuit Women

In the 1970s, Danish researchers began to study the traditional diet of Greenland natives, the Inuit. Living in the Arctic regions of Greenland (as well as Canada and Alaska), the Inuit have one of the most extreme diets on the planet. They don't farm fruits, vegetables, or grains, and there aren't many wild plants to forage. Their main source of food is what they could hunt, and they hunt mostly at sea, catching whales, seals, and fish. Despite eating so much fatty meat and fish, the Inuit don't have a lot of heart attacks, compared with individuals in more temperate countries. Plus, they suffer just one-tenth the rate of diabetes.

Later investigations revealed that the Inuit people do not have a lot of cancer, either, and there is very little breast cancer among the women. One large-scale study of the Inuit found that autoimmune diseases, such as asthma and psoriasis, are extremely rare among Inuit subsisting on fish.

What are we to make of all this? Thankfully, it has been long concluded that the omega-3 fatty acids found in fish are protective, which eventually led to the recommendation that Westerners eat more fish to help prevent these diseases. Those early investigations have stood the test of time. Mounds of other studies have reached the same conclusion: omega-3 fatty acids are vitally important to good health.

The chief reason is that these fats are highly involved in our immune system, which wards off disease, fights infection, and prevents chronic inflammation from running wild in our bodies. So it makes sense that these fats can favorably alter the course of many diseases—and even prevent them.

The diet of the Inuits is also high in vitamin D, a nutrient that keeps the bones strong by helping the body absorb calcium and phosphorus—key minerals for bone health. Menopausal Inuit women who stick to their traditional diets tend to have stronger bones than those who drift to a more Westernized style of eating, according to the research.

There's more: Inuits are known to regularly consume bone broth, which is highly alkalinizing and loaded with alkalinizing minerals. Discovering this fact through research was such an a-ha moment for me. It explained why the Inuits could thrive so well on an otherwise very acidic diet.

What we learn from the studies of Inuit populations is that foods high in omega-3 fatty acids and vitamin D, and devoid of processed foods, give us a wonderful health advantage through the years. To obtain more of these nutrients, try my Crispy Skin Salmon (page 221) and Vinegar-Poached Herby Fish (page 212).

CHAPTER 7

The Keto-Green Cleanse

The Keto-Green Cleanse is a 6-day liquid detox, designed to give your body a pause from solid food in order to work on important issues—namely, fat burning and hormone balance, boosting friendly bacteria in your gut, and strengthening your immunity. You'll forgo processed foods, sugar, and dairy; this plan is built around smoothies, various types of broth, juices, and teas.

Go on This Plan If You:

- Are feeling burned out.
- Want more energy.
- Need to lose weight, particularly belly fat.
- Struggle with food cravings.
- Desire to detox your body after a period of eating too many processed and sugar-laden foods—or consuming excessive alcohol.
- Resolve specific menopause symptoms such as fatigue, joint pain, brain fog, constipation, and skin problems such as adult acne.
- Want to fast for spiritual growth.

Women in my Keto-Green Community have nothing but praise for this cleanse. Rhonda, for example, reported that it is "easy." "I did one day of water and bone broth fasting, followed by a day of water, bone broth, and smoothies. I had no problem doing this and felt great the entire time."

Vera agreed. "I did the cleanse for five days—bone broth and smoothies. I was amazed at how easy it was."

Mary used the cleanse after a week-long eating fest over a Thanksgiving holiday: "I was with family for a week. We ate out a lot, had a sumptuous holiday dinner, cocktails most nights—the works. It was a total free-for-all in terms of food. After that week, I was terrified to get on the scale. I had achieved my goal already on Keto-Green, losing 12 pounds, and I knew I had blown it. For two days after Thanksgiving, I did a bone broth fast. Then I got on the scale. I was happily surprised—I had dropped another three pounds, below my goal weight. The cleanse is a great tool for getting back on track. I love it."

You, too, can expect many good things to happen from following this plan—and definitely within the 6 days. For proof, researchers from Thomas Jefferson University Hospital evaluated 15 healthy participants (13 women and 2 men between the ages of 21 and 85) before and after their visits to a health and wellness spa in Desert Hot Springs, California. The

Pork Bone Broth, page 240 •
Roasted Chicken Bone Broth,
page 241 • Dr. Anna's Beef
Bone Broth, page 242

week-long program included a juice fast (similar to the cleanse here), yoga, and meditation to encourage deep breathing. In other words, they paused from their usual way of eating and living.

After the data were compiled, it was clear that the program produced a number of remarkable changes. On average, people lost a pound a day, or 7 pounds in just a week. Their diastolic blood pressure—the lower of the two blood pressure measurements—decreased by 7.7 points. And hemoglobin levels in their blood increased slightly, indicating that their blood was better oxygenated. (Hemoglobin is the protein in red blood cells that transports oxygen from the lungs to the body's tissues and returns carbon dioxide from the tissues back to the lungs.)

There was also a 5.2 percent decline in cholesterol. Also, everyone felt less depressed, less anxious, and more mentally alert (a complete overturning of emotional symptoms many of us have experienced in menopause). All this in one week!

But you don't have to go to a spa to start feeling alive again. You can reset your health in the same speedy way by following this nutrient-dense cleanse. Besides the benefits like weight loss, expect to experience good things such as better digestion, quality sleep, greater energy, sharper thinking, and fewer cravings during these next 6 days.

Benefits of the Cleanse

Hormonal Balance

In one glass—I'm talking about smoothies here—you can sip a combination of nutrients that help your body get back into balance. My smoothies are packed with green leafy vegetables, low-sugar fruits, and nuts, all of which are great sources of fiber. Supplied with enough fiber, your body is able to reduce your cortisol, normalize your insulin, regulate your estrogen levels, and increase your metabolism.

Anti-inflammatory Nutrition

Foods like leafy greens contain a lot of antioxidants and phytonutrients, which help your body fight inflammation. So, when you drink smoothies and juices, you're infusing your body with a concentrated level of these nutrients.

Blueberries—a smoothie staple—also have amazing anti-inflammatory power, according to researchers from Louisiana State University. Two groups drank smoothies—with blueberries or without—twice a day for six weeks. The blueberry-infused smoothies boosted immune function, decreased free radicals, and reduced inflammation in people with metabolic syndrome, a prediabetic condition. (Blueberries have also been found to increase insulin sensitivity in obese individuals who are insulin resistant.)

Mental Clarity

With this cleanse, you're getting your body off junk food, especially processed white flour and sugar, both of which can clog your mind and make your brain feel cloudy. Drinking smoothies and bone or alkaline broths can clear your mind and focus your attention so you can think more easily.

A British study from 2019 backs me up on this. In this experiment, researchers gave 40 participants ages 20 to 30 either a smoothie containing equal amounts of blueberries, strawberries, raspberries, and blackberries, or another smoothie without these ingredients (what is called a placebo) and then put them through a series of cognitive tests. Berries like these are low-glycemic fruits, meaning they don't cause big surges in glucose and insulin.

The participants' mental performance was measured across 2 hours, 4 hours, and 6 hours. Those who drank the placebo got mentally fatigued early on and couldn't complete the tests. But those who drank the berry-infused smoothies stayed mentally sharp, with quicker response times throughout the 6 hours of testing.

Why such significant results? Berries are rich in nutrients called flavonoids, which have been shown in lots of research to exert particularly powerful actions on cognition and may even reverse age-related declines in memory and learning.

Fewer Cravings

When you pump up the nutrients in your diet with healthy vegetables, protein, and fats while staying lower in carbs and pause the processed stuff, you'll naturally stop craving junk food. You may even find yourself craving healthy food—and adding more veggies during the day after eating more nutritiously. I've seen this happen again and again. Most women I know who regularly consume smoothies and bone broth tell me the same thing: they are not hungry for *hours* after, and these foods totally shut down their sugar cravings.

Here's a little trick to make your smoothies even more satiating: blend them for about 5 minutes. This "aerates" them. In one study, incorporating air into a milkshake (through blending) so it appears twice the volume but contains the same number of calories resulted in a 12 percent reduction in food intake at the next meal, as well as lower reports of hunger.

Detoxification

Even if you commit to eating more nutritiously, there are environmental toxins working against you and invading your day-to-day life: air pollution, car fumes, the chemicals in some makeup, household cleaning products, and chemical additives in food, to name just a few. If we keep being exposed to them, these pollutants can disrupt our bodies, leading to health problems and imbalances. A proper cleanse is one way to minimize the effects of these dangers.

When you undergo a cleanse like this one, you are neutralizing and eliminating many of the toxic substances in your body.

My Cravings Cure

I've used this little secret for years with patients, clients, and in all of my women's restorative health programs. It solves cravings for processed carbs and sugary foods. The reason is that when these cravings get hold of you, it really means your body needs essential fats. In other words, you are craving carbs because your body really wants fat.

Here's how to put an end to these cravings:

Do an intermittent fast, in which you go for 15 or 16 hours between dinner and a meal the next morning.

Before that morning meal, mix ½ cup purified cod liver oil with the juice of 1 lemon or lime. It's best if the oil is cold, so remember to refrigerate it overnight. After you drink the mixture, take a bite of your lemon or lime to cut the oily aftertaste. Cheers!

Wait an hour and have your designated meal, based on the plan you're following.

I realize you may not like the idea of this cravings-stopper, but you will love how it curbs your desire to overeat, clears brain fog, and eliminates the need for white-knuckling willpower. For more information on this, see my short video on the subject at dranna.com/menupause-extras.

It will also help your body with its natural detoxification process.

Healthy Digestion

Smoothies help get things moving in the morning because they are full of prebiotics—fast food for the friendly bacteria in your gut (probiotics). When you drink a smoothie, the prebiotics from the veggies feed and support the population of good bacteria in your system and increase their diversity. This allows your gut, immune, and endocrine systems to all be in harmony.

Some amino acids present in bone broth may be helpful for digestion. One of these is glutamine. In a 2017 study, glutamine was shown to help heal the intestinal barrier in human and animal subjects. This may help with conditions such as leaky gut, in which the mucosal lining in the intestines is irritated and interferes with your body's ability to digest food.

Another study from the same year pointed out that people with inflammatory bowel disease tend to have lower levels of some amino acids in their bodies. For these people, getting additional amino acids into their diets may help with some symptoms of the condition.

The benefits of this cleanse will show up in as little as two days. Thereafter, you'll increasingly feel more energized, lighter, better rested, and experience fewer cravings and less bloating. The cleanse resets your body in a short, intense period. But I encourage you to continue eating healthfully in the future by incorporating smoothies and bone broth into your daily routine.

Pausing from Alcohol and Caffeine

The Keto-Green Cleanse can help you attain these benefits, but it is also designed to assist you in detoxing from two beverages—alcohol and caffeine—both of which can aggravate menopause symptoms.

Alcohol

Although studies have shown low to moderate alcohol consumption to be beneficial for heart health, excessive drinking can severely damage your liver function by causing fat buildup, inflammation, and scarring.

It is not necessary to swear off cocktails forever, but there are plenty of good reasons to minimize your alcohol consumption and at least keep it moderate. As defined in the most recent U.S. Dietary Guidelines, moderate drinking for women means one drink per day (or less).

Moderate means protective. Here's why. Women who have two to five drinks a day have 1.5 times the risk for breast cancer as those who don't drink at all, and heavy drinking can increase your risk for cardiovascular disease, according to the North American Menopause Society. Plus, some women find that alcohol makes them more susceptible to hot flashes.

Also, limiting or abstaining entirely from alcohol is one of the best ways to keep your body's detoxification system running strong. Doing a cleanse like this can accelerate this process and heal damaged cells.

Caffeine

Love your morning cup of joe? Me, too! But too many cups could be worsening your menopause symptoms. A Mayo Clinic study published in 2015 in the journal *Menopause* found that menopausal women who consumed caffeine were more likely to have hot flashes than women who didn't consume caffeine. Too much caffeine also triggers an upswing in cortisol and other stress hormones, which has a weight-gain effect.

As caffeinated beverages, coffee and tea are incredibly healthy, full of antioxidants and other plant chemicals that support health. However, high doses of caffeine may have other unpleasant and even dangerous side effects: anxiety, insomnia, diarrhea, high blood pressure, rapid heart rate, frequent urination, and ironically, fatigue. If any of these conditions plagues you, you might want to pause caffeine and use this plan to help you.

As much as I love coffee, taking a pause

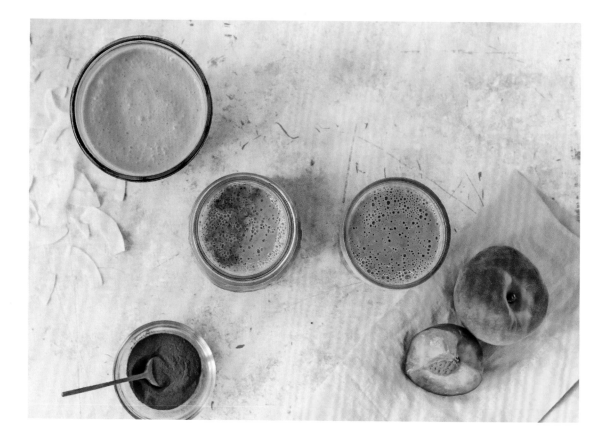

from it has been incredibly beneficial during this time of my life. What I realized was that it was creating weight-loss resistance for me and increasing my blood sugar, as well as my cortisol levels. Yes, even a single black cup of coffee can have this effect!

In the research for my book *Keto-Green 16*, I wore a continuous glucose monitor called the FreeStyle Libre for almost a year. I noticed that on mornings in which I drank coffee or my beloved espresso, my blood sugar would jump 15 to 20 points.

I was surprised, but it made sense. Caffeine is a drug that stimulates the adrenal glands to churn out lots of cortisol, which in turn increases blood sugar. The net effect of all this was to make me weight-loss resistant. I now drink coffee sparingly, and usually only after I break my fast. (See the Resources section of this book or dranna.com/menupause-extras for information on glucose monitors and testing options.)

What to Eat

The cleanse features three "meals" each day to load you with fat-burning, hormone-balancing foods. These include:

- A daily Lemon Liver Flush (page 232) to promote detoxification

- Nonstarchy greens and plant-based protein, to supply you with fiber, antioxidants, and phytonutrients

- Bone broth, to give your body healing collagen that fortifies and renews tissues

- Healthy fats, to optimize your hormones, make your brain happy, and satisfy your appetite

The Lemon Liver Flush

Upon awakening, you'll enjoy my Lemon Liver Flush (page 232). Lemons are a rich source of vitamin C, a powerful antioxidant. In fact, the juice of one lemon provides around 21 percent of the vitamin C you need daily. Vitamin C is also important for immune system function, wound healing, and helping the body absorb iron from foods. Lemons are also rich in flavonoids—anti-inflammatory compounds that help fortify health, boost brainpower, promote fat metabolism, and fight disease.

This flush is also alkalizing and promotes hydration. For information on the benefits of alkalinity, refer to page 48.

The Smoothies and Juices

With their intense infusion of nutrients, these smoothies have either kale, spinach, or another alkalinizing green as the base and then various other yummy flavors to make you feel like you're sipping a milkshake through the day—which is never a bad thing.

The juices are designed to detox your liver to improve its fat-burning and detoxification powers.

The Broths

Bone broth is made from slow boiling animal bones and connective tissue, both of which contain collagen. Cooking collagen turns it into gelatin, and that gelatin provides the body with amino acids, which are the building blocks of proteins. As I mentioned earlier, this is especially important for our bones, joints, and skin.

Bones themselves are rich in vitamins and alkalinizing minerals, including calcium, magnesium, and phosphorous, so cooking them releases these healthful components into the broth.

Pausing with Tea

One way to hydrate while cleansing, or while you are on any of these plans, is to enjoy herbal teas. Certain herbs may help balance your hormones, for example, and herbal teas made from them are a great way to reap the benefits. You may also stir a scoop of Mighty Maca Plus into any of your teas for additional hormonal support.

You can also try something called a "tea tox," in which you replace one or two meals with a cup or two of herbal tea. When I do this, or whenever I enjoy tea, I like to create a ceremony for my tea drinking, following Japanese traditions. The Japanese tea ceremony is summed up in the Zen phrase *ichi-go ichi-e*, which means "one time, one meeting." This phrase is meant to symbolize the power and beauty of the present—the "now." This moment might never come again, so give it your complete awareness and appreciation.

With a bit of awareness or mindfulness, and by simply slowing down long enough to truly enjoy it, your cup of tea can have a lasting impact on your whole day—and ultimately your spiritual path.

Here are some easy steps for creating your own tea ceremony:

1. *Select your tea.* Really, any caffeine-free tea is a perfect choice for your ceremony! Feel free to try something new or stick to your favorite. If you'd like some suggestions, refer to the chart on page 100.

2. *Brew your tea in mindfulness.* Allow it time to steep, consciously bringing your attention to the present moment. Remind yourself that this moment will never come again, so you should give it your full attention and respect. When the tea is ready, take a moment to hold the mug near your nose and just breathe in the warmth and blissful scent. Offer up the fragrance as a gift to God.

3. *Drink your tea with mindfulness—with very small sips.* Feel the warmth, taste the flavor, sense the energy, smell the aroma, and feel gratitude for this little moment of joy your cup of tea brings.

4. *Stay in the present moment.* Release whatever has happened in your life leading up to this point in time. Let go of wondering or worrying about what the future will hold. Tune in to your current state of being, then make an effort to consciously become fully present in the here and now. Remember to bring yourself back to the present whenever you find yourself mentally moving on to the next thing you might have to do today or of being pulled back into something that happened in the past.

5. *End with gratitude.* Thank the tea for sharing its leaves, beauty, and medicinal properties that gave you this calming meditation. And give thanks and appreciation for all the blessings in your life. Also, drinking tea at least three times a

week is linked with a longer and healthier life, according to a study published in the *European Journal of Preventive Cardiology*, and it is associated with lower risks of cardiovascular disease. This study included 100,902 participants with no history of heart attack, stroke, or cancer. The participants were classified into two groups: habitual tea drinkers (three or more times a week) and never or nonhabitual tea drinkers (fewer than three times a week). They were followed up for a median of 7.3 years.

This is what that study revealed: Habitual tea drinkers enjoyed more healthy years of life and they lived longer than nonhabitual tea drinkers. Habitual tea drinkers also had a 20 percent lower risk of incident heart disease and stroke, a 22 percent lower risk of fatal heart disease and stroke, and a 15 percent lower risk of all causes of death. One reason for the heart-protective quality of tea is that it is a rich source of plant polyphenols known to protect against cardiovascular disease.

The Chinese are not the only major tea drinkers in the world. The British consume 60 billion cups of tea a year, according to their Tea and Infusions Association. That's more than 900 cups a year for every man, woman, and child in Great Britain! Tea is entrenched in the British way of life, evident from the humble morning tea break to afternoon tea.

But what of its health benefits for British women who are in menopause? A study published in the *American Journal of Clinical Nutrition* reported that older women who were habitual tea drinkers had greater bone density and strength than did those who did not drink tea. The authors of the study noted that nutrients found in tea, such as flavonoids, may influence bone health and that tea drinking may protect against osteoporosis in older women.

Based on all the wonderful attributes of tea, I'd say, "Drink up"! The chart that follows lists teas that are helpful for menopause.

Top Botanical Teas for Menopause

Tea	How It Works	Best for Treating
Black cohosh	Works on serotonin in the body	Estrogen imbalance, hot flashes, and vaginal dryness
Chamomile	Contains flavonoids that are responsible for the medicinal benefits of the tea	Poor sleep quality—menstrual pain, blood sugar control, osteoporosis, and inflammation
Chasteberry	Contains flavonoids that can influence certain hormone levels in your body, especially prolactin, progesterone, and to a certain extent, estrogen	Premenstrual symptoms—particularly breast pain and soreness—and menopausal symptoms
Cranberry	Antibacterial	Urinary tract infections
Dong quai	Anti-inflammatory, anti-spasmodic	Estrogen imbalance, cramps, and menopausal pelvic pain
Elderberry	Contains an antioxidant called anthocyanin that clears the body of free radicals; also has antiviral and anti-inflammatory properties	Constipation, colds, flu, and pain
Ginger	Antioxidant, anti-inflammatory	Nausea, bloating, and gastrointestinal discomfort
Ginseng	An adaptogen that helps the body handle stress	Fatigue, hot flashes, night sweats, vaginal dryness, and hair loss
Green tea	High in phytonutrients	Fatigue and weight gain
Licorice root	Contains a compound called glycyrrhizic acid; an antioxidant, anti-inflammatory, and an anti-microbial	Stress, adrenal fatigue, cravings, skin conditions, menopause symptoms, acid reflux, and upper respiratory infections
Maca root	High in phytoestrogens, which exert a weak estrogenic effect	Libido, fatigue, and other menopausal symptoms

Tea	How It Works	Best for Treating
Milk thistle	High in phytoestrogens, which exert a weak estrogenic effect; antioxidant	Liver detoxification
Mint	High in antioxidants	Digestive issues, concentration, headaches, and hormone imbalances
Orange blossom	Sedative	Anxiety, stress, tension relief, and sleep quality
Passion flower	Sedative	Sleep disorders, night sweats, and anxiety
Red clover	High in phytoestrogens, which exert a weak estrogen effect	Estrogen imbalance, night sweats, hot flashes, bone density, high blood pressure, and immunity; and may protect against breast cancer
Red raspberry leaf	Contains fragarine, a plant compound that helps tone and tighten muscles in the pelvic area, which may reduce the menstrual cramping caused by the spasms of these muscles	Perimenopause symptoms, heavy menstrual flow, and various menopause symptoms
Rosemary	High in antioxidant, antimicrobial, and anti-inflammatory compounds	Blood sugar control, mood, memory, and brain fog
Rosewater	Hydrating, digestive support	Skin healing, relaxation, calms digestive stress
Valerian	Sedative, antispasmodic	Depression, mood swings, insomnia, and anxiety

The 6-Day Keto-Green Cleanse

For a downloadable menu plan with a graphic representation of the meals, go to dranna.com/menupause-extras.

Day 1

Upon Awakening
Lemon Liver Flush

Breakfast
Blender Green Veggie Juice

Lunch
Piña Wholada

Midday Treat
Mighty Maca Margarita

Dinner
Roasted-Garlic Bone Broth Soup OR
    Dr. Anna's Mineral Broth

Day 2

Upon Awakening
Lemon Liver Flush

Breakfast
Green Goodness Smoothie OR Pineapple-
    Pepper Green Juice

Lunch
Drinkable Berry Yogurt OR Dr. Anna's
    Mineral Broth

Midday Treat
Mighty Maca Margarita

Dinner
French-Onion Bone Broth Soup

Day 3

Upon Awakening
Lemon Liver Flush

Breakfast
Peach Melba Smoothie

Lunch
Dr. Anna's Beef Bone Broth

Midday Treat
Mighty Maca Margarita

Dinner
Dr. Anna's Mineral Broth

Day 4

Upon Awakening
Lemon Liver Flush

Breakfast
Lemon-Ginger Zinger

Lunch
Pumpkin Protein Shake OR Dr. Anna's Beef
    Bone Broth

Midday Treat
Mighty Maca Margarita

Dinner
Mediterranean Lemon Soup

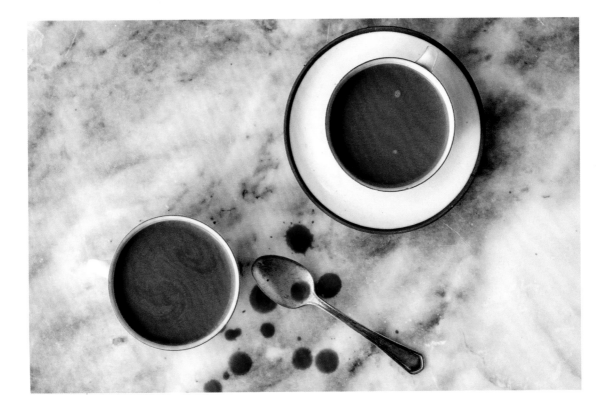

Day 5

Upon Awakening
Lemon Liver Flush

Breakfast
Nutty-for-Green Smoothie

Lunch
Creamy Vanilla–Mint Shake OR
    Dr. Anna's Beef Bone Broth OR
    Dr. Anna's Mineral Broth

Midday Treat
Mighty Maca Margarita

Dinner
Pork Bone Broth OR Dr. Anna's
    Mineral Broth

Day 6

Upon Awakening
Lemon Liver Flush

Breakfast
Collagen Hot Chocolate

Lunch
Dr. Anna's Beef Bone Broth

Midday Treat
Mighty Maca Margarita

Dinner
Pork Bone Broth OR Dr. Anna's
    Mineral Broth

Your 6-Day Shopping List

For a downloadable shopping list of this plan, go to dranna.com/menupause-extras.

Supplements and Staples to Have On Hand

Dr. Anna's Keto-Green Shake or Dr. Anna's Keto-Alkaline Protein Shake; or a good substitute protein powder that is formulated with a vegan protein such as pea or rice protein, containing less than 3 grams of sugar (per serving) and less than 10 grams of carbohydrate (per serving)

Mighty Maca Plus, 7.2-ounce container; or 1 (8-ounce) bag powdered maca root

Collagen powder, 1 (9.5-ounce) container

Probiotic capsules for yogurt, packet of 2

MCT or coconut oil, 1 (16-ounce) bottle

Extra-virgin olive oil, 1 (24-ounce) bottle

Apple cider vinegar, 1 quart bottle

Butter or ghee, 1 (8-ounce) package

Liquid stevia, 1 (1.8-ounce) bottle

Monk fruit or stevia

Vanilla extract, small bottle

Banana extract, 1 small bottle (optional because vanilla extract can be used instead)

Margarita mix (sugar-free and preferably organic), 1 (32-ounce) bottle

Cacao powder, 1 (8-ounce) package

Worcestershire sauce, 1 (10-ounce) bottle

Seasonings: sea salt, black pepper, cayenne, garlic powder

Dried herbs: parsley, sage, bay leaves

Spices: ground cinnamon, nutmeg, pumpkin pie spice, ground turmeric

Produce—Fresh Vegetables

Spinach, 6-ounce bag

Baby spinach, 6-ounce bag

Kale, 1 (6-ounce) bag

Broccoli slaw, 1 (8-ounce) package

Carrots, 9 medium

Celery, 3 bunch

Cauliflower, 1 small head

Cucumbers, 2 medium

Dandelion greens, 1 (8-ounce) package

Fresh ginger, 1 (6-inch) piece

Scallions, 1 bunch

Leek, 1 medium

Yellow onions, 4 medium, 5 large

Garlic, 3 to 4 bulbs

Mushrooms, 1 (1-pound) package

Produce—Fresh Herbs

Mint, (.5-ounce) package or 1 bunch

Parsley, 1 bunch

Rosemary, (.5-ounce) package

Thyme, (.5-ounce) package

Produce—Fresh Fruit

Avocados, 2 medium

Green apple, 1

Lemons, 19

Nuts, Nut Butters, and Seeds

Almond butter, 1 (12-ounce) jar

Cashews, unsalted, 1 (16-ounce) package

Hemp seeds or flax seeds, 1 (.5-ounce) bag

Unsweetened coconut flakes, 1 (7-ounce) bag

Protein Sources

Beef soup bones (preferably from grass-fed beef), 6½ pounds

Pork rib bones or ham hocks, 2 pounds

Chicken bones from a whole chicken or rotisserie chicken

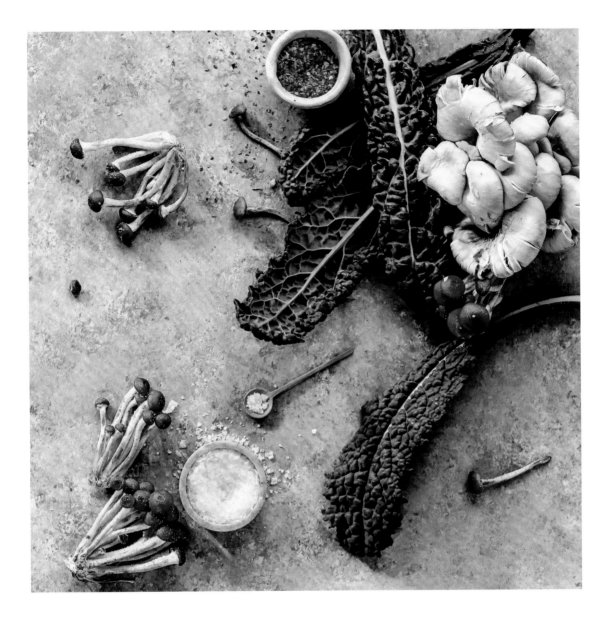

Non-Dairy Milks

Full-fat coconut milk, 1 (14-ounce) can
Unsweetend coconut milk, 1 quart
Unsweetened almond milk, 2 quarts
Unsweetened cashew milk, 1 quart
Coconut cream, 1 (14-ounce) can

Other Items

Pineapple chunks, unsweetened, ¾ cup
Pumpkin puree, 1 (15-ounce) can
Peaches, frozen, 1 (10-ounce) bag
Raspberries, frozen, 1 (10-ounce) bag
Cauliflower rice, frozen, 1 (10-ounce) bag
Coconut water, 1 (8.5-ounce) can

Strategies for Success

1. With this plan, start one day at a time. See how you feel; then gradually add another day and so forth if you are feeling good. If you take medication or are diabetic, please obtain your physician's approval prior to following this plan.

2. Focus on organic ingredients for your smoothies, juices, and broths. If you use fruits in your smoothies and juices, make sure they are low-glycemic, high-fiber, and low-sugar fruits. See the list on page 107.

3. Store your smoothies in glass bottles, if transporting.

4. Aim for variety. Try to vary your greens and your smoothies so that you are exposed to many different nutrients. Make bone broth from different types of bones, as directed.

5. Test your urinary pH and ketones first thing in the morning (and periodically throughout the day whenever you go to the bathroom), with the goal of keeping your pH at or above 7.0. The pinker the strip, the higher your level of ketosis (fat-burning). Record everything in a journal. For testing strips and journal pages, see the Resources section of this book, or go to dranna.com/menupause-extras.

6. Weigh yourself each morning so as to monitor your weight loss.

7. Hydrate! Juices and shakes contain water, and they do count as part of your liquid intake. However, the best drink you can have is plain filtered water. Drink approximately half your ideal body weight in ounces of filtered water each day. But don't drink more than 4 ounces (½ cup) of fluids with any given meal, so that your digestive juices have time to do their work. My typical recommendation is to drink water up to 20 minutes before you eat, then have 4 ounces (½ cup) of fluid with your meal, and wait one to two hours afterward.

8. Never overload your stomach. Drink your liquids until you feel full.

9. If you feel hunger pangs during the day, you can add extra healthy fats to your smoothies, or enjoy a large cup of bone broth (see pages 240–246) or a large cup of mineral broth (see page 244).

10. Even though smoothies are blended, it is still wise to sip them slowly. That way, you will feel satiated and you'll enjoy them more.

11. Don't stay on the cleanse longer than 6 days. Switch to my regular Keto-Green Plan, as outlined in *The Hormone Fix* or *Keto-Green 16*, or follow the Carbohydrate Modification Plan in Chapter 8.

Menopause Around the World: India

Women in India definitely experience the same menopause symptoms as we do in this country. But the more I delved into this topic, the more I learned. What intrigued me most is that Indian women have fewer hot flashes and night sweats than we do.

In one study, a total of 717 peri- and postmenopausal women, ages 45 to 55 years, from urban centers in different regions of India, were surveyed about their symptoms. Turns out that the prevalence of hot flashes and night sweats was low: only 34 percent of the women reported them! Those who did have hot flashes reported poorer general health and more negative beliefs about menopause (obviously how we think affects our symptoms for better or worse).

Why do Indian women have fewer hot flashes and night sweats? My feeling is that it all goes back to the traditional Indian diet, with its many high-fiber vegetables and medicinal herbs. These foods help in controlling blood sugar, for one thing, and when that is under control, hot flashes are rare.

Research now suggests that the phyto-estrogens found in fennel help manage postmenopausal symptoms and pose no adverse effects. Guess what? In India it is common to chew plain or sugar-coated fennel seeds after a meal. Fennel contains an ingredient that acts like estrogen in the body, which is why it may address various issues that crop up during menopause.

Indian cuisine also liberally uses healthful and flavorful spices and herbs like ginger, cinnamon, coriander, and turmeric, all of which are full of antioxidants and pack lots of anti-inflammatory power. The presence of lentils and chickpeas in many dishes also makes Indian food a high-fiber and vegetarian/vegan-friendly option.

You'll find many recipes in this cookbook that incorporate Indian spices. If hot flashes are one of your top complaints, here are some recipes to try: Lemon-Ginger Zinger (page 236), Fennel and Leek Pot Roast (page 154), and Coriander-Garlic Shrimp (page 275).

CHAPTER 8

The Carbohydrate Modification Plan

Here is a flexible and liberal eating plan—one that includes a variety of carbohydrates. I consider it as a feasting plan.

The basic premise of the Carbohydrate Modification Plan is to reintroduce carbohydrates into your diet. Not to worry: you will not balloon back to your old weight or gain more weight. And you will continue to look and feel as great as you do now. In fact, you will still be able to manage your menopausal symptoms.

Go on This Plan If You:

- Want to feast.
- Have successfully completed any of the other four plans and you're ready to start a maintenance plan.
- Need to ease into beneficial nutritional habits, especially if you're not ready to follow the more challenging plans.
- Have reached your desired weight and need to transition to a maintenance plan.
- Desire a more broad-based eating plan.
- Want to keep your hormones in balance, preventing the major symptoms of menopause, such as hot flashes, night sweats, sleep disturbances, fatigue, irritability and anxiety, depression, and memory problems.
- Are not carbohydrate sensitive (meaning carbs do not cause cravings or unexpected weight gain).
- Are gluten intolerant.
- Are training for a high-intensity athletic event and require a higher carb intake to fuel your training and competition.

My Carbohydrate Modification Plan offers an effortless strategy to transition from the other plans without weight gain (in fact, it can help you lose a little more) while staying alkaline and feeling in peak health. (For information on the benefits of alkalinity, refer to page 48.) Of course, the transition should be made alongside sustainable habits and lifestyle changes, such as exercise, rest, and avoidance of processed, sugary carbs and those containing gluten.

Texas Rodeo Breakfast
Skillet, page 253

Making the Switch

If you're going carb-modified after any of the other plans in this book, you've been enjoying whole, nonprocessed foods up to now, so modifying your diet to include healthy carbs is not going to feel like a big change. Here are my guidelines for transitioning to the Carbohydrate Modification Plan.

Continue the Basics of Keto-Green Nutrition

First, make organic, free-range proteins a staple of your diet (meat, poultry, fish, shellfish, and plant proteins). In fact, consider increasing them slightly. This achieves a couple of things: it helps you capitalize on the thermic effects of food (the number of calories it takes to digest food) and it helps you feel full and assists your body in adjusting more easily.

Second, stay green. Continue to eat lots of green leafy vegetables, cruciferous veggies, salad vegetables, and other low-carb, high-fiber vegetables. These have healing effects on your body and will keep it alkaline.

Third, continue eating healthy fats to combat hunger. When you start introducing carbs back into your diet, you may find that you feel hungry more often, even after meals. This can lead to overeating and weight gain. To keep unnecessary hunger at bay, make sure you continue to include healthy fats in your diet. Thus, olive oil, coconut oil, MCT oil, avocado oil, nuts, seeds, and avocados are all great sources of healthy fats.

Gradually Increase How Many Carbs You Eat

Add one to two servings of carbs for the first six days. If you're maintaining your weight, or even dropping a few pounds, continue this strategy for another six days. But if you're gaining weight, cut back to one serving for the first six days, then, add a second serving during the second set of six days.

As for grams, eat 50 to 60 grams of carbs a day for the six days, then bump that number up to 75 to 100 grams a day for another six days or for a couple days of the plan. For most people, a daily intake of about 100 grams of carbs does the trick. If the number on the scale starts inching up, cut back to the amount of carbs you ate the week before.

Select the Right Carbs

Not all carbs are equal. Bread and pasta have very few nutrients, while junk foods like doughnuts and cake have almost zero. See the following list for high-quality carbs that you should prioritize.

If you eat grains, make sure they are gluten free. Gluten is an inflammatory protein found in certain foods, mainly wheat and related grains like barley, rye, and occasionally oats. Eliminate or scale back on your gluten intake to assist in metabolism, maintain digestive health, and reduce inflammation.

When you do have fruit, choose lower-glycemic options such as seasonal berries and melons.

This is a list of carbs you can reintroduce into your diet on the Carbohydrate Modification Plan, grouped by category:

Common Legumes

The amounts given here are based on ½ cup of the cooked item. These vegetables are also good protein sources on a plant-based diet, so I've listed their protein counts as well.

Black beans—carbs: 20 grams; protein 7.5 grams

Black-eyed peas—carbs: 54 grams; protein 22 grams

Chickpeas (garbanzo beans)—carbs: 7 grams

Edamame, shelled—carbs: 10 grams; protein 16 grams

Kidney beans—carbs: 18.5 grams; protein 7.5 grams

Lentils—carbs: 20 grams; protein 9 grams

Navy beans—carbs: 27 grams; protein: 7.5 grams

Peas—carbs: 12 grams; protein: 4 grams

Pinto beans—carbs: 18 grams; protein: 7.5 grams

Split peas—carbs: 20 grams; protein: 8 grams

White beans—carbs: 29 grams; protein: 8.5 grams

Gluten-Free Grains

Amounts of carbs shown are based on ½ cup of the cooked grain.

Amaranth—23 grams
Buckwheat—17 grams
Corn—15.6 grams
Cornmeal, polenta, grits—15.5 grams
Millet—20.6 grams
Oats (gluten-free)—14 grams
Quinoa—20 grams
Rice—23 grams
Sorghum—72 grams
Teff—25 grams

Vegetables

Amounts of carbs shown are based on one medium vegetable or 1 cup of the item cooked and mashed or sliced.

Common Winter Squashes

Acorn—15 grams
Butternut—10.5 grams
Delicata—5 grams
Hubbard—11 grams
Kabocha—6 grams

Starchy Root Vegetables

Beets—2 medium beets, cooked: 10 grams; 1 cup sliced: 8.5 grams

Parsnips—1 cup: 26 grams
Potato—1 medium, baked: 37 grams
Rutabagas—1 cup: 12 grams
Sweet potato—1 medium: 24 grams
Turnip—1 cup: 8 grams

Lower-Glycemic Fresh Fruits

Apple—1 medium: 25 grams
Apricot—1 small: 3.8 grams
Blackberries—1 cup: 13.8 grams
Blueberries—1 cup: 21 grams
Cantaloupe—1 cup: 13 grams
Cherries—1 cup: 22 grams
Cranberries—1 cup: 12 grams

Figs—1 small: 8 grams
Grapes—1 cup: 16 grams
Grapefruit—1 half: 13 grams
Guava—1 medium: 8 grams
Honeydew—1 cup: 16 grams
Kiwifruit—1 medium: 10 grams
Lemon—1 medium: 5.4 grams
Lime—1 medium: 7 grams
Nectarine—1 medium: 15 grams
Orange—1 medium: 15.4 grams
Peach—1 small: 12 grams
Pear—1 medium: 27 grams
Raspberries—1 cup: 14.7 grams
Rhubarb—1 cup, cooked: 5.5 grams
Strawberries—1 cup: 12 grams
Tangerine—1 medium: 10 grams
Watermelon—1 cup: 12 grams

Pause Carbs That Are High in Sugar

Although you may be looking forward to an occasional indulgence now, it's best to avoid consuming any sugar-heavy carbs until your body has had at least two weeks to adjust. Carbs like cookies and donuts can cause your blood sugar to spike, which can make you feel tired and irritable while increasing your sugar cravings. Later on, when you have occasional feast days, you can enjoy a dessert—but don't go overboard on this.

Time Your Carbs

I recommend that you try to eat your carbohydrates at certain times of the day. On days when you exercise, you can eat your carbs before or after your workout. A number of studies have found that eating a mixed meal of carbs and protein within a few hours after a workout may help increase protein synthesis, which is the process by which your body builds metabolism-boosting muscle.

If you do resistance training, you might be better off eating the carbs beforehand. Some people find that eating carbs prior to their workouts helps them perform better. The body uses those carbs to power the workout and they will be burned off more efficiently. Maintaining a regular exercise regime will also help you avoid gaining weight as you gradually reintroduce carbs into your diet.

I recommend that you eat a carb at dinner, such as a sweet potato. Doing so helps you sleep more restfully and promotes healing rest. But does eating carbs at night make you gain weight? Not at all. In one six-month study, 78 obese adults were asked to follow a diet that involved eating carbs either only at dinner or at every meal. The dinner-only group lost more total weight and body fat and felt fuller than those who ate carbs at every meal.

Everyone is different, however. Listen to how your body feels after you reintroduce carbs into your life at different times. Stick with what feels best for you.

Once you've lost your extra weight or are ready for a dietary change, nutritious carbs can be a healthy and fun part of your diet. Follow this plan for reintroducing carbs, and you can enjoy them fearlessly, and you'll be just fine. I look forward to feast days!

The 6-Day Carbohydrate Modification Plan

For a downloadable menu plan with a graphic representation of the meals, go to dranna.com/menupause-extras.

Day 1

Breakfast
Green Chia Pudding

Lunch
Keto-Green Nachos

Dinner
Chicken with Goat Cheese, Fig Jam, and Basil AND Wild Rice Pilaf

Treat
DIY Fruit Parfait

Day 2

Breakfast
Bacon 'n' Egg Bundles

Lunch
Leftover Chicken with Goat Cheese, Fig Jam, and Basil OR
Brussels Me Up Salad

Dinner
Pan-Seared Coriander Lamb Chops, served with a side of brown rice or a baked potato

Treat
Gluten-Free Chocolate Chip Cookies

Day 3

Breakfast
Texas Rodeo Breakfast Skillet

Lunch
Country Ham and White Bean Soup with Mustard Greens

Dinner
Za'atar-Roasted Salmon with Garlicky Bean Mash AND Anytime Keto-Green Salad

Treat
Lemon Panna Cotta

Day 4

Breakfast
Baby Kale Breakfast Salad with Smoked Salmon and Avocado

Lunch
Salmon Quinoa Bowl

Dinner
Country Ranch Meatloaf

Treat
Riesling Poached Pears

Day 5

Breakfast
Poached Eggs on Swiss Chard

Lunch

Tarragon Chicken Salad with Apples and
Pecans

Dinner

Leftover Country Ranch Meatloaf

Treat

Vanilla and Fig Scones with Pistachios

Day 6

Breakfast

Shakshuka

Lunch

Twice-Baked Sweet Potatoes AND Brussels
Me Up Salad

Dinner

Coriander-Garlic Shrimp

Treat

Keto Almond Delight

The DIY Meal Option

In addition to using the recipes, you can
build your own meals by following a simple
template:

Breakfast = 1 protein serving + 1 vegetable
+ 1 fat serving.

An example would be 2 scrambled eggs,
1 cup greens, and some sliced avocado.

Lunch = 1 protein serving + 1 vegetable
+ 1 serving of a permissible carb + 1 fat
serving.

An example would be 1 pan-fried ground
beef patty + 1 cup greens sautéed in
1 tablespoon olive oil or coconut oil +
1 serving of cooked quinoa.

Dinner = 1 protein serving + 1 serving
vegetables + 1 serving a permissible carb (if
not eaten at lunch) + 1 fat serving.

An example would be 1 baked chicken thigh
+ mashed sweet potatoes + a side salad
with fresh greens tossed with 1 tablespoon
olive oil and lemon juice.

Your 6-Day Shopping List

For a downloadable shopping list of this
plan, go to dranna.com/menupause-extras.

Supplements and Staples to Have On Hand

Mighty Maca Plus, 7.2-ounce container; or
    1 (8-ounce) bag powdered maca root
Nutritional yeast, 1 (5-ounce) package
Extra-virgin olive oil, 1 (16-ounce) bottle
Coconut oil, 1 (14-ounce) jar
Avocado oil, 1 (16-ounce) bottle
Balsamic vinegar (sugar-free), 1 (16-ounce)
    bottle
Red wine vinegar, 1 (16-ounce) bottle
Dry white wine, 1 (750 ml) bottle
Riesling wine, 1 (750 ml) bottle (or other
    fruity white wine)
Vegenaise, 1 (15-ounce) jar
Ghee, 1 (13-ounce) jar (optional)
Butter, 1 (8-ounce) package

Liquid stevia, 1 (1.8-ounce) bottle

Erythritol, 8 ounces

Coconut sugar, 1 (1-pound) bag

Maple syrup, 1 (12.5-ounce) bottle

Raw honey, 1 (16-ounce) jar

Organic cane sugar, 1 (1-pound) bag

Vanilla extract, small bottle

Vanilla beans, 2 whole

Almond extract, small bottle

Cacao powder, 1 (8-ounce) package

Baking soda

Unflavored gelatin, 1 (1-ounce) box

Almond flour, 1 (32-ounce) bag

Minced garlic, 1 (4.5-ounce) jar

Capers, 1 (3.5-ounce) jar

Spicy brown mustard, 1 (12-ounce) jar

Sriracha sauce, 1 (9-ounce) bottle

Seasonings: sea salt, black pepper, black peppercorns, lemon pepper seasoning, paprika, red pepper flakes, onion powder, garlic powder

Spices: ground cumin, ground turmeric, ground coriander, coriander seeds, cinnamon sticks, whole cloves

Dried herbs: tarragon, thyme or za'atar blend, chives, dill, sage, rosemary

Produce—Fresh Vegetables

Spinach, 8 ounces

Kale, 2 (16-ounce) bags

Mustard greens, 1 (16-ounce) bag

Rainbow Swiss chard, 1 (1-pound) bunch

Arugula, 1 (16-ounce) bag

Mixed baby greens, 1 (16-ounce) bag

Carrot, 1 medium

Celery, 1 bunch

Cucumber, 1 medium

Brussels sprouts, 8 ounces, shaved

Radishes, small bunch

Bean sprouts, 1 (4-ounce) package

Fresh ginger root, 1 (4-inch) piece

1 serrano pepper

Yellow onions, 6 medium

Red onion, 1 large

Bell pepper, any color, 1

Green bell pepper, 1

Garlic, 2 bulbs

Sweet potatoes, 1 small, 2 medium

Tomatoes, 2 large, 2 medium, 2 small

Zucchini, 1 large

Mushrooms, 1 (8-ounce) package

Produce—Fresh Herbs

Basil, 1 (.5-ounce) package or 1 bunch

Cilantro, 1 bunch

Mint, 1 (.5-ounce) package or 1 bunch

Parsley, 1 bunch

Rosemary, 1 (.5-ounce) package

Sage, 1 (.5-ounce) package

Thyme, 1 (.5-ounce) package

Produce—Fresh Fruits

Avocados, 3, medium

Lemons, 10

Apple, 1 small

Lime, 1

Orange, 1 navel

Pears, 2 medium

Selected berries, 1 pint: blueberries, strawberries, raspberries, blackberries

Nuts, Nut Butters, and Seeds

Almonds, slivered, 1 (10-ounce) bag

Almonds, sliced, 1 (10-ounce) bag

Almonds, whole, 1 (8-ounce) bag

Cashews, raw, 1 (16-ounce) package

Pecans, chopped, 1 (8-ounce) bag

Pistachios, shelled, 1 (24-ounce) bag
Pine nuts, 1 (8-ounce) bag
Chia seeds, 1 (12-ounce) bag
Coconut flakes (unsweetened), 2 (7-ounce) bags
Sunflower seeds, 1 (16-ounce) bag

Protein Sources
Eggs, large, 1½ dozen
Salmon, 1 (6-ounce) can (preferably wild-caught)
Salmon, smoked, 1 (6-ounce) package
Salmon fillets, 4 (4- to 6-ounces each)
Shrimp, fresh, 7 ounces
Chicken breasts, 2 boneless, skinless, 6 to 8 ounces each
Baked chicken breasts, 2 boneless, skinless, and shredded to make 1 cup
Chicken cutlets, 2 thin, 4 ounces each
Turkey, ground, 1½ pounds (not ultra-lean)
Lamb rib chops, 6 per person
Country ham, sliced, 8 ounces
Bacon (no sugar), 1 (8-ounce) package
Pork breakfast sausage, ground, ½ pound
Shrimp, 7 ounces, peeled and deveined

Grains
Brown rice, long-grain, 1 (1-pound) bag
Quinoa, 1 (16-ounce) bag
Wild rice, 1 (8-ounce) box

Non-Dairy Milks and Milk Products
Unsweetened almond milk, 1 quart
Full-fat coconut milk, 3 or 4 (14-ounce) cans
Coconut cream whip, 1 (8-ounce) carton
Coconut cream, 3 (14-ounce) cans

Other Items
Jam of choice, 1 (8-ounce) jar (Adriatic fig spread or apricot or raspberry jam)
Cheese, goat (chèvre), 1 (4-ounce) log
Kidney beans, 1 (16-ounce) can
Great Northern or cannellini beans, 1 (16-ounce) can
Tomatoes, diced, with green chilies, 1 (14-ounce) can
Dried figs, 1 (8-ounce) container
Kalamata olives, pitted, 1 (6.5-ounce) jar
Salsa of choice, 1 (24-ounce) jar
Chicken broth, 1 (32-ounce) can
Guacamole, store-made 1 (15-ounce) carton
Cacao nibs, 1 (8-ounce) bag
Chocolate chips, 1 (8-ounce) bag, 100% or 85% cacao
Stevia dark chocolate chips, 1 (9-ounce) package
Cauliflower rice, frozen, 1 or 2 (10-ounce) packages
Tomato sauce, 1 (8-ounce) can

Menopause Around the World: Italy

I love Italian food, especially pasta. However, I enjoy it only when I do my occasional feast. One reason to put that pasta fork down is that a diet with too much pasta and other refined carbs, like white rice, has been linked to an increase in insulin resistance in women. This condition can cause problems with the body's levels of hormones, such as estrogen, resulting in earlier menopause and frequent hot flashes.

Which brings me to Italian women. Pasta is a staple in Italy, so how do they handle menopause?

Pretty easily, according to the research. Surveys show that Italian women are less likely to think of menopause as something bad or as an end to the prime of their lives. They view menopause positively, as a normal phase of life they must pass through. Nearly 40 percent of Italian women believe that menopause is a good experience for a woman.

Women in Italy are the least likely to report vaginal dryness, hot flashes, and night sweats as menopause symptoms and are more likely to say that menopause was a much better experience than they had anticipated.

A huge reason why Italian women have positive menopause experiences is their Mediterranean-style diet. It's packed with fish, vegetables, fruits, nuts, legumes, whole grains, and olive oil—all of which have anti-inflammatory and antioxidant actions. Because of these benefits, many studies have shown that the Mediterranean diet is heart protective and also associated with a reduced risk of breast cancer. And an important note: when Italian women do eat pasta—which is frequently—it is in much smaller portions than Americans might consider standard. Intermittent religious fasting is also a part of their culture.

For a taste of Italy, try these *MenuPause* dishes: Rainbow Mediterranean Salad (page 131), Stovetop Ratatouille (page 193), and Lemon Panna Cotta (page 280).

Strategies for Success

1. Follow this plan exactly as written or substitute any meal with DIY meals you create based on the food lists.

2. You have the option of intermittent fasting on this plan. This type of fasting condenses your entire food intake to a specific window of time. A popular way to begin this is 16 hours of fasting and 8 hours of feeding, or 16:8. So, for example, if you have your last meal at 6:00 p.m., you wouldn't eat the next day until after 10:00 a.m. And, yes, sleeping time counts toward fasting! Intermittent fasting helps with weight loss, reduced inflammation, cellular renewal, detoxification, and other conditions.

   Alternatively, you may feel that you require only two meals daily in an 8-hour eating window, and find just two meals satisfying. This is an effective way to eat, because it encourages weight loss and maintenance.

3. Test your urinary pH first thing in the morning and your ketones (and periodically throughout the day whenever you go to the bathroom), with the goal of keeping your pH at or above 7.0. As for ketones, the pinker the strip, the higher your level of ketosis (fat-burning). Record everything in a journal.

4. Weigh yourself each morning so as to monitor whether you are gaining, losing, or maintaining weight.

5. Hydrate! Drink approximately half your ideal body weight in ounces of filtered water each day. But don't drink more than 4 ounces (½ cup) of fluids with any given meal, so that your digestive juices have time to do their work. My typical recommendation is to drink water up to 20 minutes before you eat, then have 4 ounces (½ cup) of fluid with your meal, and wait one to two hours afterward.

6. Never overload your stomach. When you begin to feel full, stop eating.

7. The treats are optional. It's preferable to not eat between meals. If you're over 40, snacking can be destructive to your goals. It can cause insulin resistance, weight gain, hot flashes, and inflammation. If you feel hunger pangs during the day, sip a cup of bone broth or mineral broth. Or. you can add more healthy fats and oils to green leafy salads.

8. Keep your carb grams at or within recommended limits.

9. You can stay on the Carbohydrate Modification Plan indefinitely, especially as a maintenance tool. If you find yourself gaining weight, return to one of the other plans in this book until you return to your happy weight.

Opposite: DIY Summer Fruit Parfait, page 279

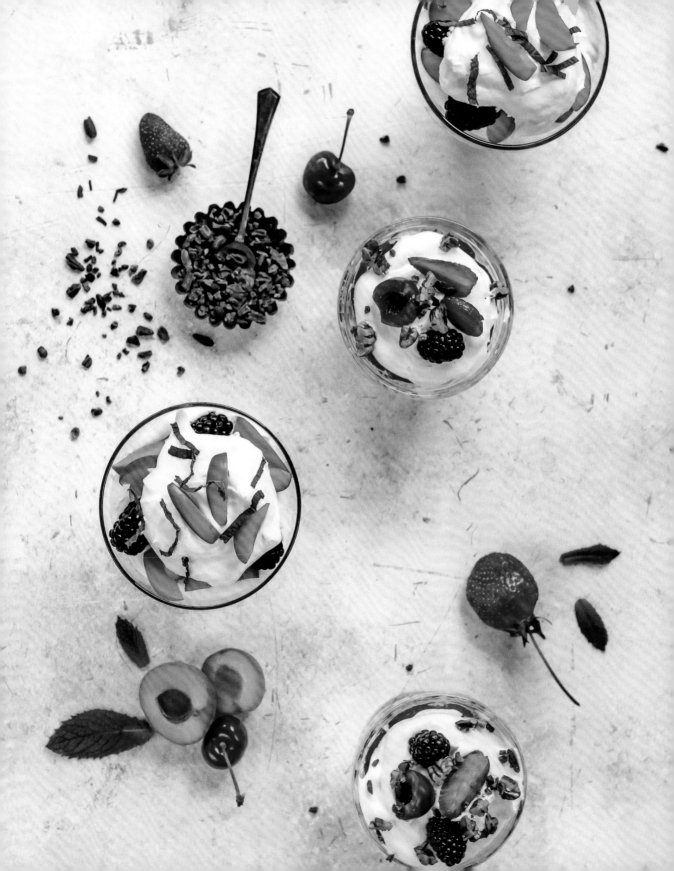

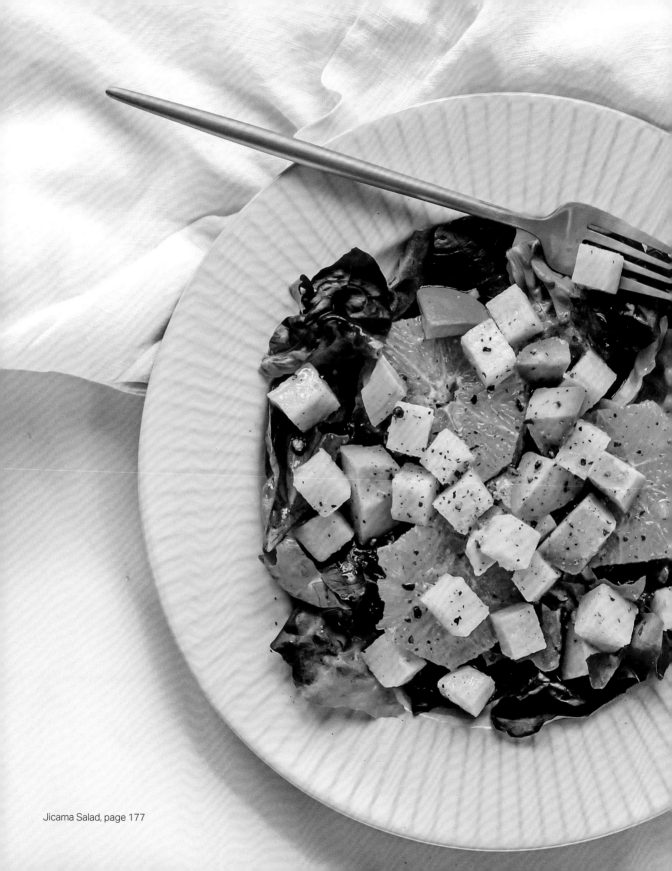

Jicama Salad, page 177

PART 3

The *MenuPause* Recipes

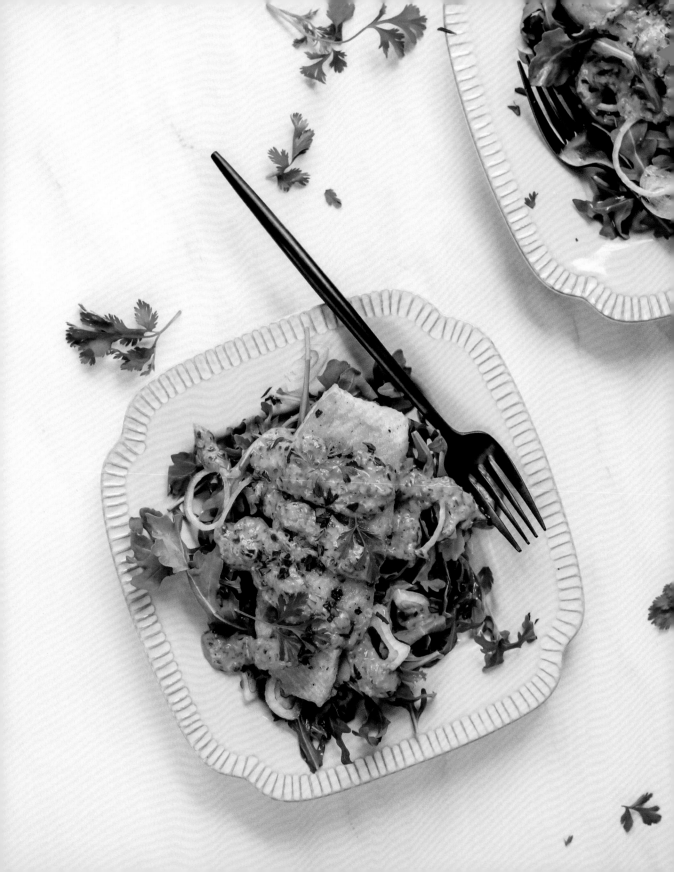

CHAPTER 9

Keto-Green Extreme Recipes

To view videos of the preparations for some of these recipes, go to dranna.com/menupause-extras.

* These recipes can be used in other plans as well. See the recipe pages for more information.

Dr. Anna's Basic Keto-Green Meal Replacement Shake MAKES 1 SERVING

1 to 2 scoops Dr. Anna's Keto-Green Shake or Dr. Anna's Keto-Alkaline Protein Shake (see Note)

1 tablespoon MCT or coconut oil, or ½ avocado (optional)

2 scoops Mighty Maca Plus, or 1 teaspoon maca root powder

1 cup water

The base for this yummy shake is a blend of pure vegan protein and nutritious plant extracts, including maca. It also contains healthy fats to support ketosis and hormone production. The blend helps you pump up your intake of green veggies by way of a delicious alkalinizing shake.

Place all the ingredients in a blender and blend well. If you prefer a very cold or thicker shake, blend in ½ cup crushed ice.

NOTE: Or substitute protein powder; it should be formulated with a vegan protein such as pea or rice protein or collagen protein and contain less than 3 grams of sugar (per serving) and less than 10 grams of carbohydrate (per serving).

NOTE: This recipe can also be used on the Keto-Green Plant-Based Detox Plan.

Extreme Green Smoothie

MAKES 1 SERVING

- 1 scoop Dr. Anna's Keto-Green Shake mix (see Note)
- 1 scoop collagen powder
- 1 tablespoon MCT or coconut oil
- 1 handful fresh spinach or other greens
- 1 cup frozen unsweetened blueberries or ¼ avocado
- 2 scoops Mighty Maca Plus, or 1 teaspoon maca root powder
- ½ cup water
- ½ cup unsweetened almond milk

Fortify your body first thing in the morning with collagen powder for healthy skin and joints, alkalinizing foods like greens and maca (terrific for balancing your hormones), and the phytonutrients found in blueberries. This smoothie can help kick-start your day, for sure!

Place all the ingredients in a blender and blend well.

NOTE: Or substitute protein powder; it should be formulated with a vegan protein such as pea or rice protein or collagen protein and contain less than 3 grams of sugar (per serving) and less than 10 grams of carbohydrate (per serving).

Good Morning Farmer's Breakfast Casserole MAKES 2 SERVINGS

1 tablespoon avocado oil

8 ounces grass-fed ground beef

1 medium onion, diced

2 cups chopped fresh spinach or kale

Sea salt

1 cup small cauliflower florets

½ cup chilled canned coconut milk, scooped from the top of the can

1 tablespoon chopped fresh parsley (for garnish)

Sometimes, you want something hearty in the morning, right? This dish serves up heartiness in a big way, plus it offers a combo of alkalinizing and detoxifying veggies. Compounds such as the DIM (diindolylmethane) and indole-3-carbinole (I3C) in cruciferous vegetables like kale and cauliflower help metabolize and break down excess estrogens in the body for healthy hormone balance during menopause.

Preheat the oven to 400°F. Grease a small baking dish with the avocado oil.

In a medium nonstick skillet, brown the beef and onion, 5 to 8 minutes. Add spinach or kale. Sauté another 1 to 2 minutes. Season to taste with the salt, then transfer to a medium bowl.

In a blender or food processor, puree the cauliflower and the coconut cream. Add this mixture to the bowl with the beef and onion, and mix well. Season with extra salt, if desired. Transfer to the prepared baking dish and bake for 35 minutes, until warmed through.

Garnish with parsley prior to serving.

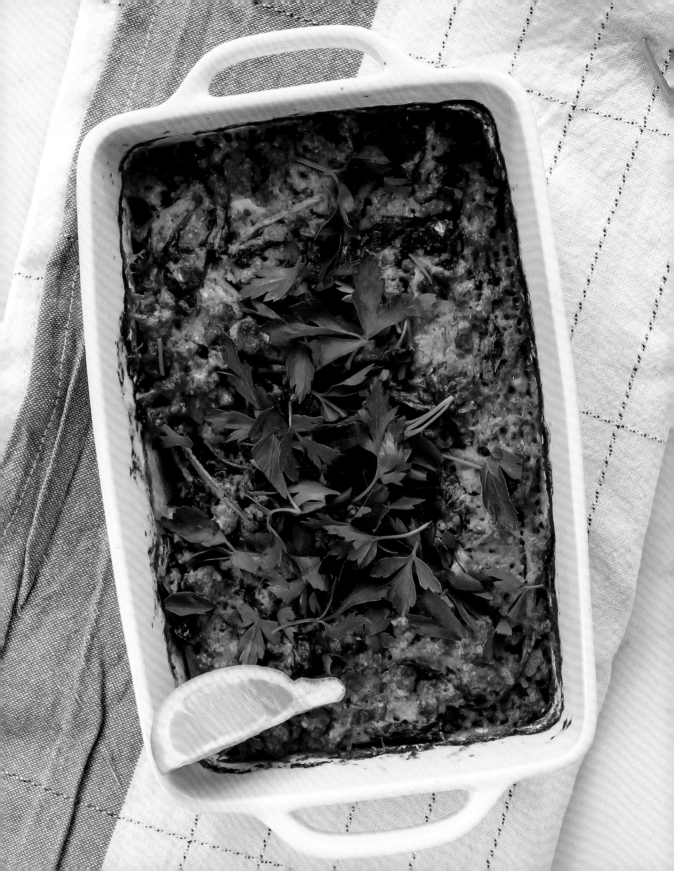

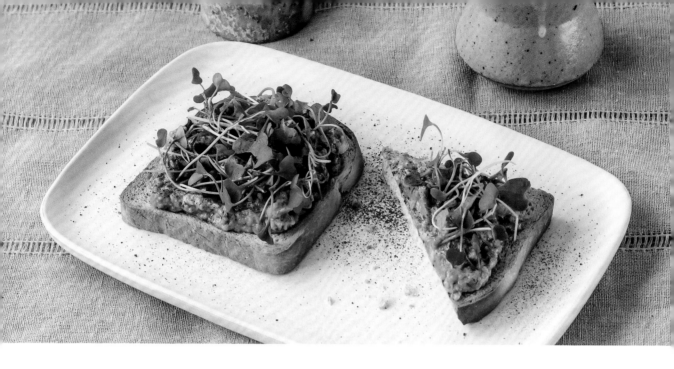

Avocado Veggie Toast   MAKES 2 SERVINGS

1 **avocado**

2 **teaspoons fresh lemon juice**

2 **tablespoons finely chopped fresh spinach or other greens, plus some for garnish**

1 **tablespoon extra-virgin olive oil**

¼ **teaspoon garlic powder**

¼ **teaspoon sea salt**

2 **slices Casabi Artisan Flatbread or 2 slices of bread made from AIP Rustic Bread Mix, both available from Amazon, or serve on large, firm lettuce leaves**

Pinch of turmeric

This toast is not only big on flavor but also takes just minutes to prepare. That kind of efficiency counts when you are busy in the morning. Avocado not only is rich in many nutrients but also promotes estrogen production (which declines in our menopausal years).

Mash the avocado in a small bowl. Add the lemon juice, the 2 tablespoons spinach, the olive oil, garlic powder, and salt. Blend into a paste.

Toast the bread, then spread with the avocado mixture. Sprinkle with turmeric and garnish with chopped spinach or other greens. Alternatively, skip the toast and serve with permitted vegetables.

NOTE: This recipe can also be used on the Keto-Green Plant-Based Detox and the Carbohydrate Modification Plan.

Smoked Salmon Breakfast Tower

MAKES 2 SERVINGS

½ cup fresh spinach or other greens

1 (3-ounce) package sliced smoked salmon, wild-caught

1 avocado, sliced

¼ cup thin red onion slices

2 tablespoons drained capers

Sea salt

Extra-virgin olive oil

To me, smoked salmon is a delicious choice for breakfast. It's loaded with omega-3 fatty acids, for starters. In 2019, a study suggested that omega-3 fat helps reduce the frequency of hot flashes and other symptoms related to menopause. The greens and avocado here boost the dish's alkalinity. Flavored with classics like red onion and capers, the salmon and greens are a breakfast winner.

Arrange the greens on 2 salad plates. Place the salmon slices on top, followed by the avocado slices. Garnish with the onion slices and capers. Taste for seasoning and add salt. Drizzle with olive oil and serve.

Warm Mushroom Salad MAKES 2 SERVINGS

- ¼ **cup extra-virgin olive oil, plus more for greasing the baking dish**
- 4 **portobello mushrooms**
  Sea salt
- 1 **tablespoon no-sugar balsamic vinegar**
- 1 **tablespoon chopped fresh basil**
- 1 **tablespoon minced fresh parsley**
- 1 **teaspoon minced garlic**
- 2 **scallions (white and green parts), sliced**
- 6 **Romaine lettuce leaves**

Portobello mushrooms are prized for their meaty taste and texture, and they make a wonderful vegan dish. They're also high in fiber and minerals. Don't forget that mushrooms are an excellent source of vitamin D, an essential nutrient that plays a role in the production and biological activity of many of our hormones.

Preheat the oven to 350°F. Lightly coat a small baking dish with a bit of the olive oil.

Slice the mushrooms into bite-size pieces or leave them whole. Salt lightly, then arrange in the prepared baking dish. Whole mushrooms should be roasted underside up. Bake for 15 to 20 minutes, until the mushrooms are roasted through.

Meanwhile, prepare the dressing. Combine the ¼ cup olive oil, vinegar, basil, parsley, garlic, and scallions. Whisk until well combined.

Place the lettuce leaves (3 per serving) on 2 salad plates, add the mushrooms, and drizzle with the dressing.

NOTE: This recipe can also be used on the Keto-Green Plant-Based Detox and the Carbohydrate Modification Plan.

Garlic-Roasted Asparagus

MAKES 2 SERVINGS

½ to 1 bunch fresh asparagus

1 tablespoon extra-virgin olive oil

1 teaspoon minced or crushed garlic

Sea salt

Juice of 1 lemon

Did you know that asparagus has the reputation of being an aphrodisiac? Rich in folate, B vitamins, and histamines (which are part of your body's defense system), this super-veggie can help you get into the mood.

Preheat the oven to 400°F.

Wash the asparagus and trim the tough bottoms. Place in a medium bowl and toss with the olive oil, garlic, and salt to taste.

Arrange the asparagus on a baking sheet in a single layer. Roast for 8 to 10 minutes, until the asparagus is tender yet crisp. Squeeze the lemon juice over the asparagus and serve.

NOTE: This recipe can also be used on the Keto-Green Plant-Based Detox and the Carbohydrate Modification Plan.

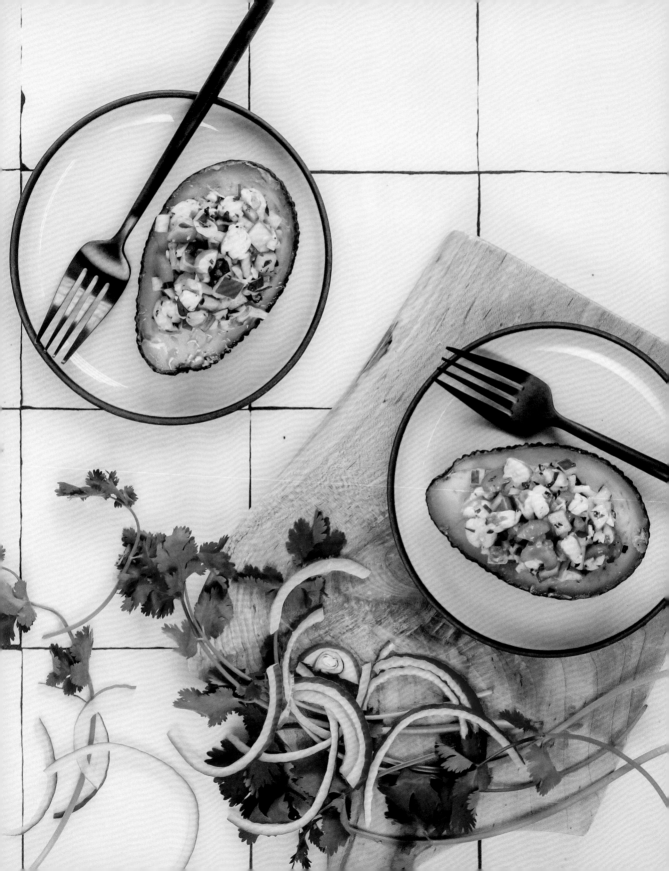

Coastal Lime Shrimp and Avocado Salad MAKES 2 SERVINGS

2 tablespoons extra-virgin olive oil

2 teaspoons apple cider vinegar

1 tablespoon chopped fresh cilantro

1 celery stalk, chopped

¼ cup chopped red onion

12 ounces jumbo shrimp, peeled, deveined, and cooked

Sea salt

1 large avocado

Lime wedges

Coming from coastal Georgia, where I had my first medical practice, I got to know many hard-working shrimpers. They knew how much I love shrimp, and occasionally I'd walk into my office and find a bag of fresh shrimp awaiting me—a gift from a grateful client. It was one of the great perks of living in a small town where shrimping is the main industry.

In a medium bowl, combine the olive oil, vinegar, cilantro, celery, and red onion. Mix well.

Chop the shrimp into small pieces and add to the dressing. Season to taste with salt.

Slice the avocado in half lengthwise and remove the pit, but do not peel. Spoon the shrimp salad into the avocado halves. Squeeze a wedge of lime over each avocado and serve immediately.

NOTE: This recipe can also be used on the Carbohydrate Modification Plan. Feel free to add a carbohydrate as a side dish.

Tuna and Celery Hand Salad

MAKES 2 SERVINGS

2 (5-ounce) cans tuna, drained and flaked

3 celery stalks, chopped

2 scallions (white and green parts), chopped

1 avocado, cubed

1 tablespoon chopped fresh dill

2 tablespoons MCT or extra-virgin olive oil

1½ tablespoons fresh lemon juice

Sea salt

2 large sturdy Romaine or Bibb lettuce leaves

1 radish, thinly sliced

2 tablespoons chopped fresh parsley

2 tablespoons chopped celery leaves (if available)

Who doesn't love a good tuna salad? Here it is, packed with a variety of veggies that pair beautifully with the omega-3–loaded tuna. You scoop the tuna salad into lettuce leaves, which substitute for bread, and eat this dish like a wrap.

In a large bowl, combine the tuna, celery, scallions, avocado, dill, olive oil, and lemon juice. Season to taste with salt. Place the lettuce leaves on 2 plates and top with the tuna mix. Garnish with the radish slices, parsley, and celery leaves, then fold up like a wrap.

NOTE: This recipe can also be used on the Carbohydrate Modification Plan. Feel free to add a carbohydrate as a side dish.

Rainbow Mediterranean Salad

MAKES 2 SERVINGS

4 Persian cucumbers, or 1 English cucumber

I cup finely chopped red cabbage

3 tablespoons finely chopped fresh parsley

3 tablespoons finely chopped fresh mint

3 tablespoons extra-virgin olive oil

Juice of 1 lemon

Sea salt

1 teaspoon to 1 tablespoon (to taste) dried sumac (a tangy spice of Middle Eastern cuisine, but optional)

I grew up eating a lot of Middle Eastern and Mediterranean meals, in which salads are an integral part, along with "mezza," which are small dishes that are shared (like tapas). This salad brings together both cultures. Plus, it is super colorful, like a rainbow, which means that it is filled with health-building phytonutrients.

Slice the cucumbers in half lengthwise and use a teaspoon to scoop out and discard the seeds. Chop the cucumbers into ¼-inch pieces. Place the cucumbers and the cabbage in a large bowl.

In a small bowl, whisk together the parsley, mint, olive oil, lemon juice, salt to taste, and sumac. Pour the dressing over the cucumbers and cabbage, and then serve.

NOTE: This recipe can also be used on the Keto-Green Plant-Based Detox and Carbohydrate Modification Plan. Feel free to add a carbohydrate as a side dish.

Dr. Anna's Cauliflower and Leek Soup

MAKES 2 SERVINGS

1 large leek, cut in half lengthwise, washed thoroughly

1 head cauliflower

2 tablespoons extra-virgin olive oil

4 cups chicken or vegetable broth

Sea salt

One evening, I had planned to make cauliflower soup for a dinner party. The number of guests increased unexpectedly, and I didn't have enough cauliflower for the soup, so I had to improvise. Fortunately, I had some gorgeous leeks on hand, so I added those. What a delicious combo! Plus, leeks are a member of the onion family, which offers nourishing benefits for your skin, hair, and overall health.

Slice all the white and some of the green of the leek. Chop the cauliflower, including the core. Heat the olive oil in a large soup pot over medium-high heat, add the leek, and sauté for about 5 minutes, until soft. Add the cauliflower, cover, and sauté for another 5 to 10 minutes.

Add the broth and bring to a boil. Reduce the heat to low and simmer for about 40 minutes, until the cauliflower is soft. Transfer the soup to a blender and blend until smooth (or use an immersion blender right in the pot). Season to taste with salt and serve. (This soup freezes well, plus it makes a delicious leftover for the next day.)

NOTE: This recipe can also be used on the Keto-Green Plant-Based Detox (made with vegetable broth) and the Carbohydrate Modification Plan. Feel free to add a carbohydrate as a side dish.

Cauli Rice with Veggies

MAKES 2 SERVINGS

- 2 tablespoons extra-virgin olive oil
- 1 medium carrot, chopped
- ½ cup sliced button or baby bella mushrooms
- 1 medium onion, chopped
- 2 cups frozen cauliflower rice, cooked according to package directions
- 2 tablespoons coconut aminos
- 1 teaspoon celery flakes
- 2 teaspoons dried parsley
- 1 teaspoon sea salt

I'm absolutely crazy about cauliflower rice, the "grain look-alike" that can be swapped for rice in many traditional recipes, thereby slashing the carb count considerably. Plus, as a detoxifying vegetable, cauliflower is a much healthier alternative to the starchy rice. You can chop a head of cauliflower yourself to make the rice, but it's more convenient to buy the frozen prepared rice in the grocery store.

Heat the olive oil in a large skillet over medium-high heat. Add the carrots and cover. Cook for 4 minutes without stirring. Remove the lid, stir, and add the mushrooms and onion. Cook for another 4 minutes or until all the vegetables are tender.

Lower heat to medium. Add in the cauliflower rice, coconut aminos, celery flakes, parsley, and salt. Stir to combine. Cook until mixture is heated throughout.

NOTE: This recipe can also be used on the Keto-Green Plant-Based Detox and Carbohydrate Modification Plan. Feel free to add a carbohydrate as a side dish or make it with cooked brown rice.

Egg Roll Soup Bowl SERVES 2

2 tablespoons extra-virgin olive oil

8 ounces ground pork

Sea salt

4 garlic cloves, chopped

1 small onion, chopped

1 small head green cabbage, cored and chopped

⅓ cup shredded carrot

1 tablespoon grated fresh ginger

3 tablespoons coconut aminos

3 to 4 cups chicken broth or bone broth

2 scallions (white and green parts), chopped

You know all those yummy, meaty fillings in Chinese egg rolls? Well, here they are, delicious as ever, in a bowl instead. Cabbage is one of the cruciferous veggies that is a good food choice when you're going through menopause. Not only does it help protect against breast cancer and heart disease, but it also is loaded with nutrients that support bone health, such as calcium, magnesium, and folic acid. (There are no eggs in this recipe, though, because it is a Keto-Green Extreme dish.) This soup can be made on the stovetop but is also conveniently made in a slow cooker.

Stovetop Directions

Heat the olive oil in a large pot over medium-high heat. When oil is hot, add the pork and season with salt. Cook for about 10 minutes, until the meat begins to brown and is nearly cooked through. Use a slotted spoon to transfer it to a bowl.

Add the garlic and onion to the hot oil and cook, stirring, for 2 to 3 minutes, until the onion begins to soften and become translucent. Add the cabbage, carrot, and ginger to the pot. Stir and cook for another 3 to 4 minutes, until the vegetables start to grow tender.

Seasoning to taste with salt as you cook, add the coconut aminos and start adding the broth to the pot, beginning with 3 cups and adding more until

(recipe continues)

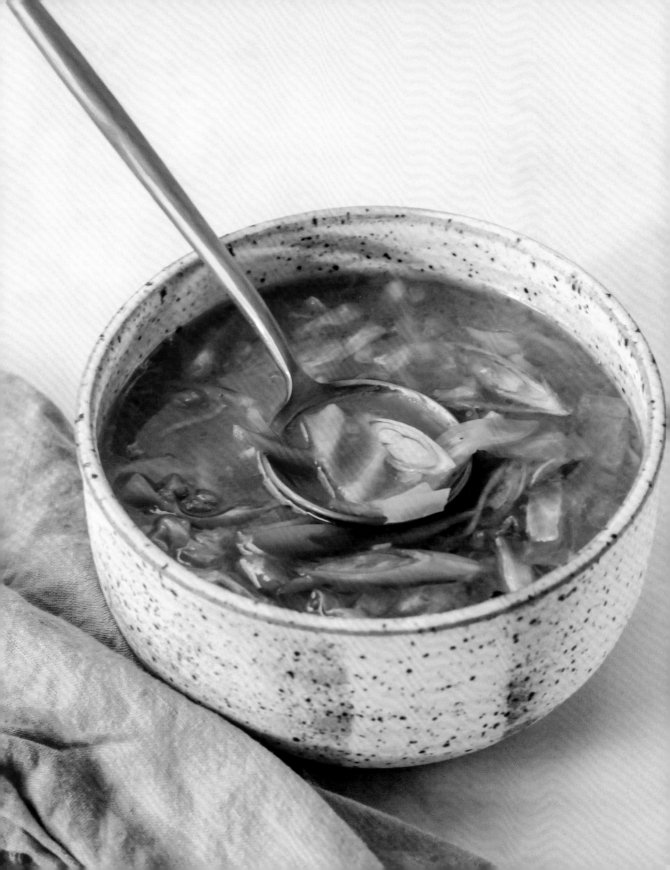

ingredients are covered. Return the pork to the pot and bring to a boil, then reduce the heat to medium-low and simmer for 25 to 30 minutes. Spoon the soup into bowls and garnish with the scallions.

Slow Cooker Directions

Heat the olive oil in a large skillet over medium-high heat until hot and shimmering, then add the pork. Cook until the meat begins to brown, then add the garlic and season with salt. Cook for another 2 minutes, then transfer to a slow cooker.

Add the onion, cabbage, carrots, ginger, and coconut aminos to the slow cooker. Start adding 3 cups of broth and continue until ingredients are covered. Close the cooker and set to cook on high for 3 to 4 hours. When ready to serve, open the cooker and spoon into bowls, then garnish with the scallions.

NOTE: This recipe can also be used on the Carbohydrate Modification Plan. Feel free to add a carbohydrate as a side dish.

Greek Keto-Green Salad

2 cups chopped kale or mixed greens

1 English cucumber, seeded and diced

½ cup chopped red onion

½ cup pitted Kalamata olives

2 tablespoons extra-virgin olive oil

2 tablespoons apple cider vinegar

¼ teaspoon onion powder

1 teaspoon dried parsley

½ teaspoon dried thyme or za'atar (a thyme spice blend)

½ teaspoon dried oregano

¼ teaspoon sea salt

Here's one of my go-to salads for staying Keto-Green. It features all the mainstays of Greek cooking—olives, cucumbers, and Mediterranean spices. I like to use apple cider vinegar in recipes as much as possible; its natural antioxidant properties help flush the body of toxins. Additionally, the vinegar alkalinizes the body.

Place the kale, cucumber, red onion, and olives in a medium bowl.

Whisk together the olive oil, vinegar, onion powder, parsley, thyme, oregano, and salt to taste in a small bowl. Pour the dressing over the salad and toss well.

NOTE: This recipe can also be used on the Keto-Green Plant-Based Detox and Carbohydrate Modification Plan. Feel free to add a carbohydrate as a side dish.

Warm Spinach and Kale Salad with Bacon and Basil Thyme Vinaigrette

MAKES 2 SERVINGS

- 4 slices (no-sugar) bacon
- 1 small onion, chopped
- ¼ teaspoon sea salt
- 1 cup baby spinach
- 1 cup baby kale
- 4 tablespoons Basil Thyme Vinaigrette (recipe follows)

Ah, bacon—one of its greatest uses is as a flavoring. It is both salty and savory, with a little bit of smokiness. Nutritionally, bacon delivers many high-quality vitamins and minerals. It is a source of saturated fat, which our bodies require for hormone production. I especially love bacon in salads like this one.

Arrange the bacon strips in a small skillet over medium heat and cook for 5 minutes, until slightly crisp. Set the bacon on paper towels to drain, then pour off half the fat in the pan.

Add the onion and salt to the skillet and cook over medium-low heat for 20 minutes, stirring occasionally. Roughly chop the bacon, then return it to the pan just long enough to reheat it.

Place the spinach and kale in a bowl and toss with the vinaigrette. Spoon the hot onion and bacon over and serve. Optional: You can sauté the spinach and kale slightly if you have digestive issues or suffer bloating.

NOTE: This recipe can also be used on the Carbohydrate Modification Plan. Feel free to add a carbohydrate as a side dish.

Basil Thyme Vinaigrette

MAKES 1 CUP DRESSING

½ cup sugar-free balsamic vinegar

2 teaspoons Dijon mustard

3 garlic cloves

¼ cup fresh basil leaves

2 fresh thyme sprigs

⅔ cup extra-virgin olive oil

Place the vinegar, mustard, garlic, basil, and thyme in a blender or small food processor and puree until smooth. With the blender running, slowly pour in the oil in a steady stream.

Continue blending for 15 seconds to fully incorporate the oil. (Alternatively, you can finely mince the garlic and whisk it together with other ingredients, then slowly whisk in the olive oil until emulsified.)

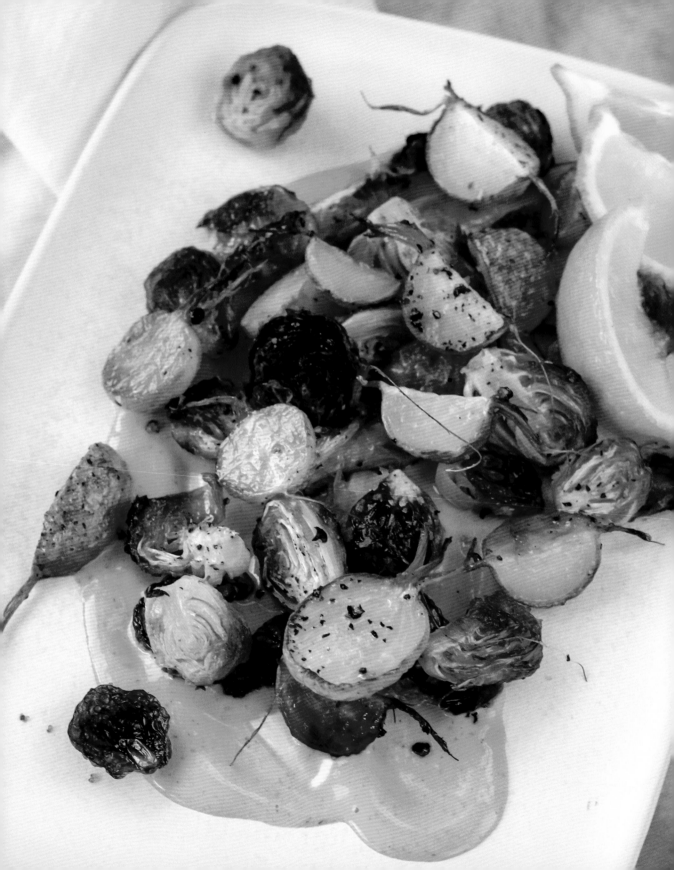

Roasted Brussels Sprouts with Radishes

MAKES 2 SERVINGS

8 ounces radishes (about a handful)

1 pound fresh Brussels sprouts, trimmed and sliced into thirds

2 tablespoons extra-virgin olive oil

½ teaspoon sea salt

Juice of ½ lemon

Here is a combination of roasted vegetables that is sure to become a favorite side dish on your dinner table. Roasted Brussels sprouts are delicious on their own, but add radishes to them and the taste goes off the charts. Roasting the radishes transforms them into a sweet and buttery veggie. Like Brussels sprouts, radishes are a cruciferous vegetable that helps detoxify harmful substances in the body.

Preheat the oven to 450°F.

Cut the radishes into roughly the same size. Place in a large bowl and add the Brussels sprouts.

Drizzle the olive oil over the vegetables and then sprinkle with the salt. Toss to coat everything well with the oil.

Spread the vegetables on a baking sheet. Roast for 18 minutes, until crisp-tender and the Brussels sprouts start to brown. Transfer the veggies to a shallow dish, then drizzle with the lemon juice and serve immediately.

NOTE: This recipe can also be used on the Keto-Green Plant-Based Detox and Carbohydrate Modification Plan.

Lemony Broccoli MAKES 2 SERVINGS

2 cups sliced broccoli florets

2 tablespoons extra-virgin olive oil

1 teaspoon dried Italian seasoning

Grated zest and juice of ½ lemon

¼ teaspoon sea salt

Broccoli has a long, impressive résumé of health benefits. It is high in many nutrients, including fiber, vitamin C, vitamin K, iron, and potassium. It also boasts more protein than most other vegetables. I love the fact that it is a terrific detoxifier, not to mention that this veggie just tastes so delicious in the right recipes, like this one.

In a medium pot, steam the broccoli for 3 to 5 minutes, until tender but still firm. Transfer to a serving bowl.

In a small saucepan over medium-low heat, combine the olive oil, Italian seasoning, lemon zest and juice, and salt. Cook for 2 minutes. Toss the broccoli with the dressing and serve.

NOTE: This recipe can also be used on the Keto-Green Plant-Based Detox and Carbohydrate Modification Plan.

ENTREES

Keto-Green Tom Kha Gai MAKES 2 SERVINGS

2 to 3 tablespoons coconut oil (for stovetop cooking)

1½ cups shiitake mushrooms, trimmed and sliced

1 tablespoon minced lemongrass

1 tablespoon grated fresh ginger

3 garlic cloves, chopped

1 medium onion, halved and sliced

Sea salt

⅓ cup shredded carrot

2½ cups chicken or beef bone broth

2 kaffir lime leaves

8 ounces boneless, skinless chicken thighs, cut into strips

1 (14-ounce) can full-fat coconut milk

2 cups chopped fresh spinach

¼ cup chopped fresh cilantro

Here's another traditional Thai dish, also known as coconut chicken soup. It is one of the most popular soups in Thailand, and one of the most popular in my household, too. Plus, it is another dish loaded with phytonutrients to help decrease menopause symptoms. This can be made on the stovetop or in a slow cooker.

Stovetop Directions

Heat 2 tablespoons of the coconut oil in a large pot over medium-high heat. When oil is hot, add the mushrooms and cook for 3 to 4 minutes, until golden on the edges. Use a slotted spoon to transfer to a bowl.

If the pot seems dry, add another tablespoon coconut oil. Then add the lemongrass, ginger, garlic, and onion. Stir, season with salt, and cook for about 2 minutes. Add the broth and kaffir lime leaves.

As soon as the broth comes to a boil, reduce the heat to medium-low and add the chicken. Stir the chicken to separate in the broth and cook for 6 to 7 minutes, until cooked through.

(recipe continues)

2 scallions (white and green parts), sliced

8 fresh basil leaves, sliced

½ lime, cut into wedges

Add the mushrooms back to the pot along with the coconut milk and spinach. Stir and cook for another 10 to 15 minutes, then remove and discard the kaffir lime leaves. Taste and adjust the salt as needed. Spoon into bowls and serve with the cilantro, scallions, and basil on top, and lime wedges on the side.

Slow Cooker Directions

In a slow cooker, combine the mushrooms, lemongrass, ginger, garlic, onion, salt, broth, kaffir lime leaves, and chicken. Cover the slow cooker and set to cook on high for 2½ to 3 hours.

When ready to serve, uncover and stir in the coconut milk and spinach, then cover again and cook for 15 to 20 minutes. Uncover, taste, and adjust salt as needed. Discard the kaffir lime leaves. Serve in bowls with the cilantro, scallions, and basil on top, and lime wedges on the side.

NOTE: This recipe can also be used on the Carbohydrate Modification Plan. Try serving it with cooked brown rice.

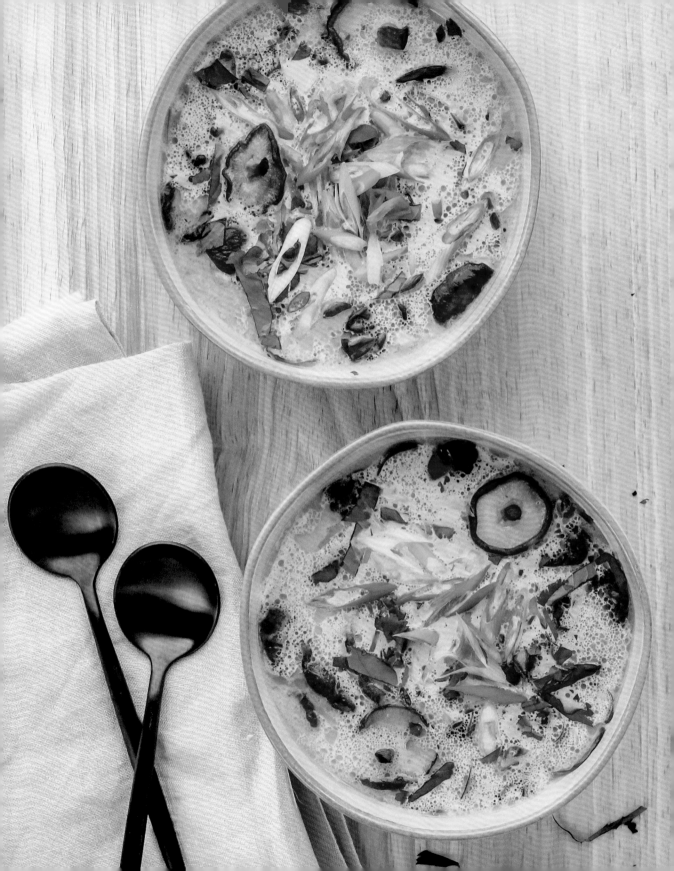

Georgia Buffalo Shepherd's Pie

MAKES 2 SERVINGS

For the filling

1 tablespoon extra-virgin olive oil

8 ounces ground beef or bison

Sea salt

1 medium onion, chopped

4 garlic cloves, chopped

1 teaspoon chopped fresh oregano

½ teaspoon chopped fresh thyme

1 large carrot, chopped

2 cups chopped green cabbage

1 tablespoon apple cider vinegar

2 tablespoons coconut aminos

2½ cups beef broth or bone broth

For the topping

3 cups small cauliflower florets, steamed until soft

1 cup diced celeriac, steamed until soft

½ cup full-fat canned coconut milk

1 tablespoon nutritional yeast

Sea salt

Shepherd's pie is a preparation that dates back to the 1800s, when housewives in Scotland were looking for ways to use leftover lamb and vegetables. Traditionally, it's topped with a layer of mashed potatoes, but here mashed cauliflower (delicious and detoxifying) substitutes so as to downsize the carbs.

Make the filling. Heat the olive oil in a large skillet over medium-high heat. Add the meat, season lightly with salt, and cook for 2 minutes, until beginning to brown. Add the onion and garlic and cook for another 2 minutes, then transfer the mixture to a slow cooker.

Add the herbs, carrot, cabbage, vinegar, coconut aminos, and broth to the slow cooker. Stir to combine and adjust the salt and pepper to taste.

Make the topping. In a food processor or blender, combine the steamed cauliflower and celeriac with the coconut milk, nutritional yeast, and salt to taste. Blend until smooth.

Spread the cauliflower and celeriac puree over the meat and veggies in the slow cooker, then cover and set the cooker on high for 3 to 4 hours. When ready to serve, open the cooker and spoon out the servings onto plates.

NOTE: This recipe can also be used on the Carbohydrate Modification Plan. Try topping it with mashed sweet potatoes in place of the mashed cauliflower.

Oven-Poached Salmon with Zesty Lemony Slaw

MAKES 2 SERVINGS

2 salmon fillets, 4 to 6 ounces each, skin removed

1 tablespoon olive oil

Sea salt

2 large lemons, 1 sliced and 1 juiced

1 small red onion, halved and sliced

⅓ cup chicken or beef bone broth

1 teaspoon chopped fresh dill

1½ tablespoons drained capers

Zesty Lemon Slaw (recipe follows)

Gently poaching these salmon fillets in the oven (or slow cooker) is a delicious, nutritious way to prepare a dish that is high in omega-3 fats for weight control, heart health, and an easier menopause. The oven-poaching preserves the moisture in the fish while adding more flavor from the broth and lemon juice. And the slaw goes so well with it, matching the lemony flavor—yummy! To make this the ultimate in easy preparation, it can be made in the oven or in a slow cooker.

Oven Directions

Preheat the oven to 325°F.

Lightly coat the fillets on both sides with the olive oil and season with salt. Arrange the lemon and red onion slices on the bottom of a medium baking dish. Pour the lemon juice and broth into the dish, then arrange the salmon on top of the slices. Sprinkle with the dill and capers.

Cover the baking dish with parchment paper and bake for 20 to 25 minutes, until the fish flakes easily with a fork. Unwrap and transfer the fillets to plates. Serve with the slaw.

(recipe continues)

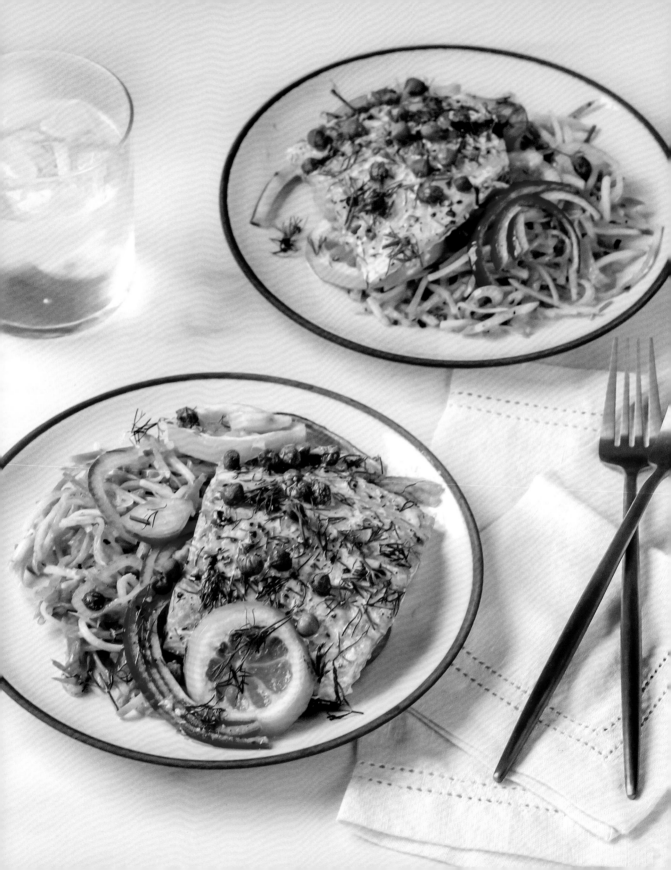

Slow Cooker Directions

Place a folded sheet of parchment paper on the bottom of the slow cooker. Arrange the lemon slices and red onion slices on top of the parchment, then pour the lemon juice and broth over. Arrange the salmon fillets on top of the lemon slices and season with the dill and the salt and pepper. Scatter the capers on top.

Cover the slow cooker and set to cook on low for 1½ to 2 hours, until the salmon flakes easily with a fork. Uncover and transfer the salmon fillets to plates. Serve with the slaw.

Zesty Lemony Slaw

MAKES ABOUT 2½ CUPS

2½ cups broccoli slaw

1 small shallot, thinly sliced

Grated zest and juice of 1 lemon

3 tablespoons extra-virgin olive or MCT oil

Sea salt

In a medium bowl, combine the slaw, shallot, lemon zest and juice, olive oil, and salt. Toss together, taste and adjust salt as needed, and let sit for at least 30 minutes to meld the flavors. I like to pour any additional juice over the salmon too!

NOTE: This recipe can also be used on the Carbohydrate Modification Plan. Feel free to add a carbohydrate as a side.

Asian Zoodle Pad Thai

MAKES 2 SERVINGS

2 tablespoons coconut oil

8 ounces thin chicken cutlets

Sea salt

1 medium onion, halved and sliced

¼ cup shredded carrot

1½ cups chopped red cabbage

4 baby bok choy, sliced lengthwise

1 large zucchini, cut into thin ribbons (spiralized, if possible)

2 tablespoons coconut aminos

½ cup bean sprouts

¼ cup chopped fresh cilantro

½ lime, cut into wedges

Traditionally, pad Thai is a stir-fried rice-noodle dish from Thailand. Here, I've used many of its traditional ingredients and spices, but have cut the carbs, substituting bean sprouts and shredded cabbage for the noodles and adding lots of extra veggies. There are phytonutrients in this dish; women who consume phytonutrients have very few hot flashes and other menopausal symptoms.

Heat 1 tablespoon of the coconut oil in a large wok or large skillet over medium-high heat. Add the chicken and season with salt, then cook for 5 to 6 minutes, until cooked through. Remove from the wok and set aside.

Add remaining tablespoon coconut oil to the wok, and when it melts, add the onion and carrot. Cook for 3 minutes, then add the cabbage. Cook for another 2 minutes, then add the bok choy and zucchini. Return the chicken to the wok, season with the coconut aminos, then adjust with salt as needed. Cook for 3 to 4 minutes, until the bok choy wilts and the zucchini strips are tender.

To serve, spoon onto plates and top with the bean sprouts and cilantro. Place the lime wedges alongside, for squeezing on top.

NOTE: This recipe can also be used on the Carbohydrate Modification Plan. Try serving it with cooked brown rice.

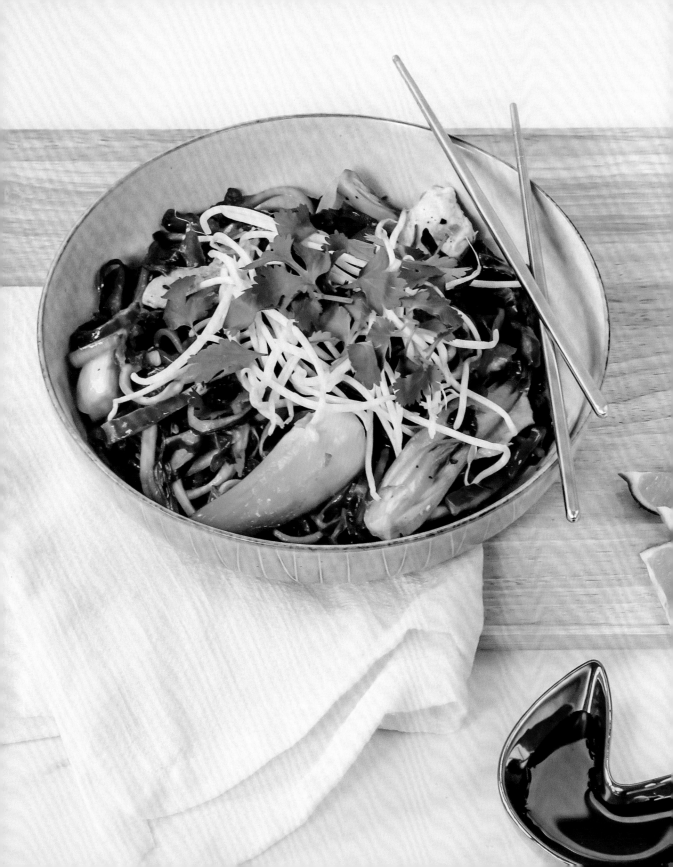

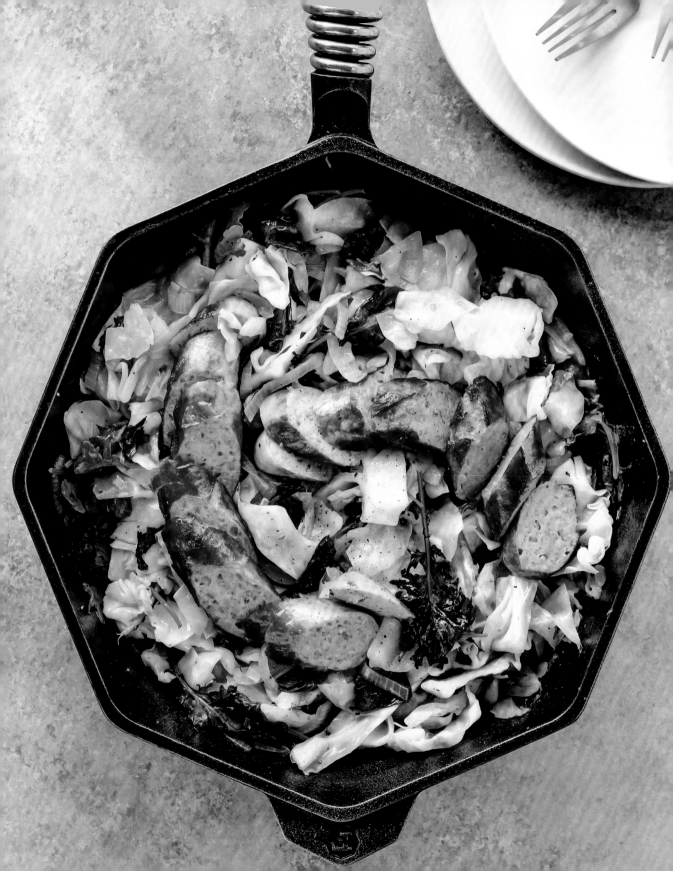

Cabbage and Kale Bratwurst Skillet MAKES 2 SERVINGS

2 organic bratwurst sausages, such as Organic Prairie

2 tablespoons olive oil

1 medium onion, halved and sliced

4 garlic cloves, chopped

½ small head green cabbage, cored and chopped

Sea salt

3 cups baby kale

2 tablespoons apple cider vinegar

Looking for a way to cook kale because you've heard that it's a superfood? Look no further than this dish. Kale is super-yummy when matched up with spicy, smoky bratwurst. Add the cabbage (a frequent partner of bratwurst), onions, and garlic, and you've got a delicious, filling meal everyone will love.

Heat a large skillet over medium-high heat. When hot, add the bratwurst and cook for 8 to 10 minutes, until heated through, rotating it to brown on all sides. Transfer to a plate.

Add the olive oil to the skillet and reduce the heat to medium. Add the onion and garlic, and cook for about 3 minutes, until the onion just begins to become translucent. Add the cabbage and cook for 5 minutes, until wilted and tender. Season to taste with salt.

Add the kale and vinegar to the skillet, stirring to combine. Slice the bratwurst and return to the skillet. Cook for another 2 minutes or until the kale wilts, then serve.

NOTE: This recipe can also be used on the Carbohydrate Modification Plan. Feel free to add a carbohydrate as a side dish.

Fennel and Leek Pot Roast MAKES 2 SERVINGS

2 tablespoons extra-virgin olive oil

1 pound boneless beef chuck roast

Sea salt

1 leek, trimmed and sliced

4 garlic cloves, chopped

2 fennel bulbs, trimmed, cored, and chopped

1 large shallot, chopped

2 cups beef broth or beef bone broth

2 tablespoons apple cider vinegar

3 fresh oregano sprigs

2 fresh thyme sprigs

1 bay leaf

Indigenous to the Mediterranean region and used extensively in Indian cuisine, fennel is an anise-flavored flowering plant that is a member of the carrot family; the bulb, fronds, and seeds are all edible. Research published in *Menopause*, the journal of the North American Menopause Society (NAMS), suggests that the phytoestrogens found in fennel help manage postmenopausal symptoms and pose no adverse effects. Here, fennel bulbs are combined with leeks and shallots to form a bed for the chuck roast in this hearty, filling dish. The dish can be prepared on the stovetop or in a slow cooker.

Stovetop Directions

Heat the olive oil in a large Dutch oven over medium-high heat. Season both sides of the beef with salt, then sear on both sides until lightly browned, about 1 minute per side. Transfer the meat to a plate.

Add the leek, garlic, fennel, and shallot to the Dutch oven. Season with salt and cook, stirring, for 5 to 8 minutes, until softened and the garlic begins to turn golden brown.

Return the meat to the pot and add the broth, vinegar, oregano, thyme, and bay leaf. When the broth begins to simmer, reduce the heat to its lowest setting and cover the pot. Cook for 3 to 4 hours, until the meat is tender and breaks apart easily with a fork. Discard bay leaf and woody herbs before serving.

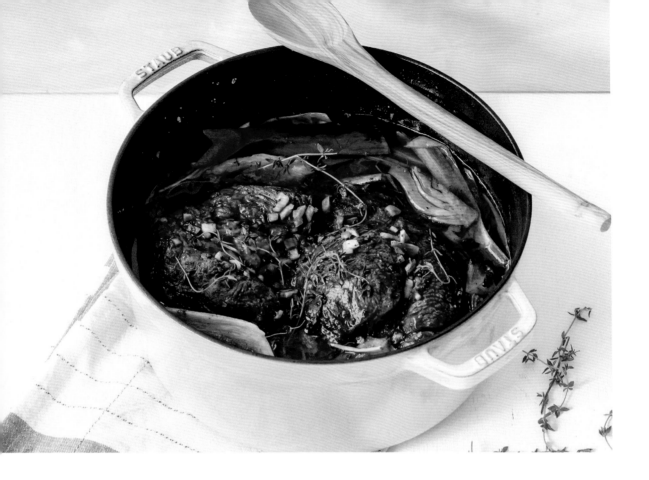

Slow Cooker Directions

Heat the oil in a large skillet over high heat. Season both sides of the meat with salt, then sear on both sides of beef until lightly browned, about 1 minute per side.

Put the leek, garlic, fennel, and shallot in a slow cooker. Place the beef on top, then pour in the broth and vinegar. Add the herbs and bay leaf. Cover the slow cooker and set to cook on high heat for 4 hours. Uncover, remove and discard the bay leaf and herb sprigs, then serve.

NOTE: This recipe can also be used on the Carbohydrate Modification Plan. Feel free to add a carbohydrate as a side dish.

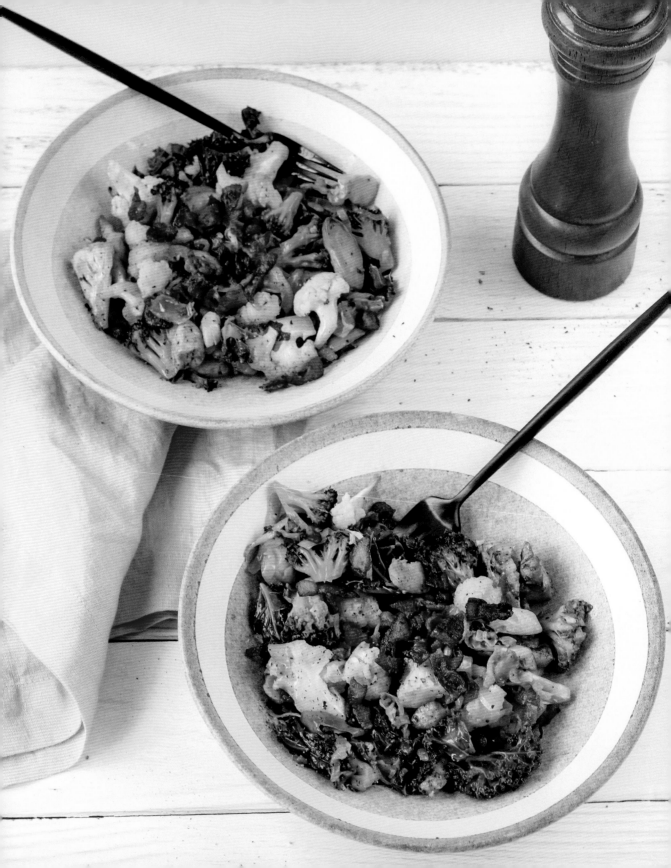

Chicken and Bacon Cruciferous Stir-Fry
MAKES 2 SERVINGS

4 slices (no-sugar) bacon, chopped

6 ounces boneless, skinless chicken thighs, cut into strips

Sea salt

1 to 2 tablespoons olive oil, as needed

1 small onion, halved and sliced

4 garlic cloves, chopped

1 cup small cauliflower florets

1 cup small broccoli florets

1 cup shredded fresh Brussels sprouts

2 cups stemmed and chopped fresh kale

Juice of 1 lemon

Packed with my favorite Keto-Green veggies, this stir-fry takes advantage of the smokiness of bacon and the juiciness of chicken thighs. Making a stir-fry like this is a quick and easy way to prepare a balanced, healthy, and delicious meal. Also, there are four different cruciferous veggies in this recipe for detoxification and hormonal support.

Heat a large nonstick skillet over medium-high heat. When the skillet is hot, add the bacon and cook to preferred doneness, chewy or crispy. Remove with a slotted spoon and transfer to a plate lined with a paper towel.

Add the chicken to the skillet and season lightly with salt. Cook for 5 to 6 minutes, until cooked through. Remove from the skillet and set aside with the bacon.

If the skillet is dry, add the tablespoon or so of olive oil, then add the onion and garlic, and cook for about 4 minutes, until the onion is translucent. Add the cauliflower and broccoli, seasoning with salt as you stir it in. Cook the cauliflower and broccoli for about 5 minutes, then add the Brussels sprouts. Cook for 2 more minutes, until the sprouts are tender. Stir in the kale and lemon juice. Cook another 3 to 4 minutes, until the kale has wilted. Add the chicken and bacon, stir to blend, then serve.

NOTE: This recipe can also be used on the Carbohydrate Modification Plan. Serve it with cooked brown rice on the side.

Halibut with Arugula Salad and Avocado Chimichurri

MAKES 2 SERVINGS

4 cups arugula or other leafy green

1 medium shallot, thinly sliced

3 tablespoons white wine vinegar

¼ cup extra-virgin olive or MCT oil

Sea salt

2 tablespoons coconut oil

2 pieces halibut fillet, 4 to 6 ounces each

Avocado Chimichurri (recipe follows)

My mouth waters when I read this recipe, mainly because I love all the greens in it. Halibut is a great fish to cook (not to mention one of the richest sources of the antioxidant, anti-aging mineral, selenium) and is very versatile. It tends to be expensive; if unavailable, you can substitute any firm white fish fillet.

In a large bowl, combine the arugula, shallot, vinegar, and olive oil. Season lightly with salt. Spread the arugula salad on serving plates.

Heat the coconut oil in large skillet over medium-high heat. Season both sides of the fish with salt, then sauté the fish in the skillet for 3 to 4 minutes per side, until the fish flakes easily with a fork.

Transfer the fish fillets to the plates with the salad and serve with a generous drizzle of chimichurri.

NOTE: This recipe can also be used on the Carbohydrate Modification Plan. Feel free to add a carbohydrate as a side dish.

Avocado Chimichurri

MAKES ABOUT ½ CUP

½ cup chopped fresh parsley

½ cup chopped fresh cilantro

½ avocado, cubed

2 garlic cloves

1 small shallot

Juice of 1 lemon, or more as needed

1 tablespoon red wine vinegar, or more as needed

2 tablespoons extra-virgin olive oil

Sea salt

In a blender, combine all the ingredients, adding a pinch of salt. Blend until smooth. If the sauce is too thick, add a bit more vinegar or lemon juice. Adjust the flavor by adding salt, if needed.

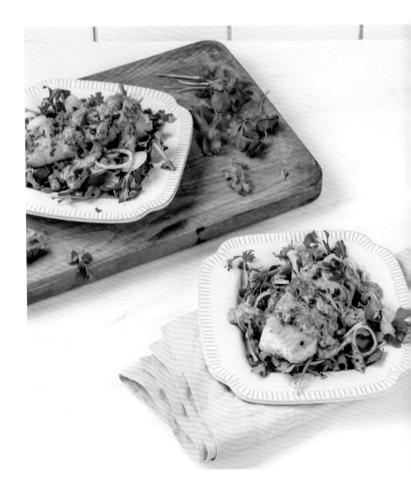

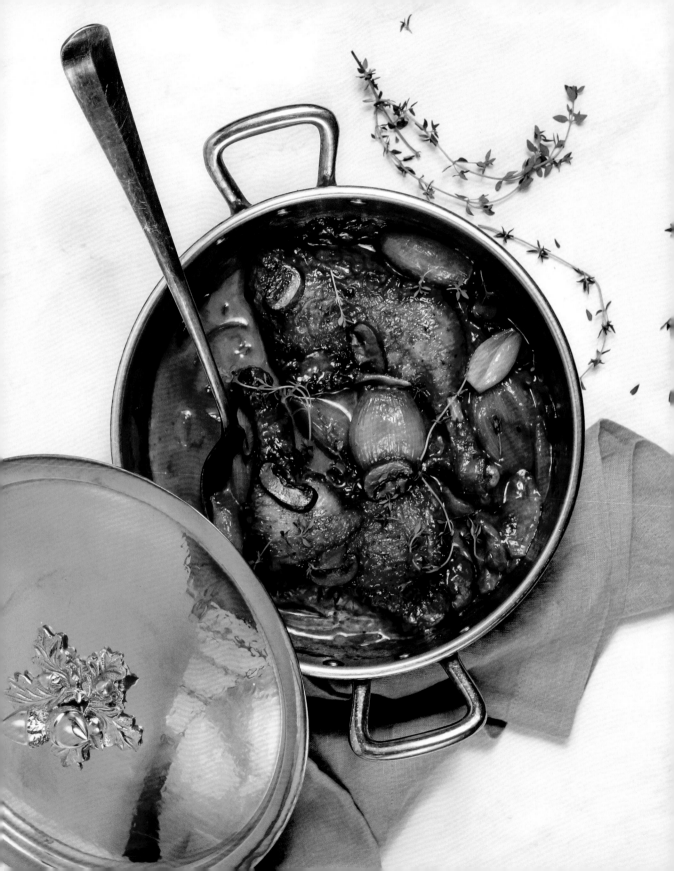

Mom's Coq au Vin

MAKES 2 SERVINGS

¼ cup extra-virgin olive oil

2 bone-in, skin-on chicken thighs (about 8 ounces total)

2 bone-in, skin-on chicken drumsticks (about 8 ounces total)

Sea salt

1 cup dry red wine*

8 to 10 shallots or small onions

1 cup sliced button or baby bella mushrooms

2 garlic cloves, crushed

*The alcohol cooks off.

Here is a family favorite from my childhood. I've made it Keto-Green, yet it's just as delicious as the traditional way that my mom prepared it. My family loves this version, and I frequently make it for dinner parties. Still, when I make it the aromas fondly take me back to my mother's kitchen.

Pour the olive oil into a large frying pan and place over medium-high heat. Season the chicken with some salt. When the oil is hot, add the chicken to the pan and brown on all sides, about 10 minutes.

Pour the wine over the chicken in the pan, then add the shallots, mushrooms, and garlic. Cover the pan with a lid, turn the heat down to low, and simmer until the chicken is tender, about 20 minutes.

Transfer the chicken to serving plates, and spoon some of pan juices over. As Mom would say, "Bon Appétit!"

NOTE: This recipe can also be used on the Carbohydrate Modification Plan. Feel free to add a carbohydrate as a side dish.

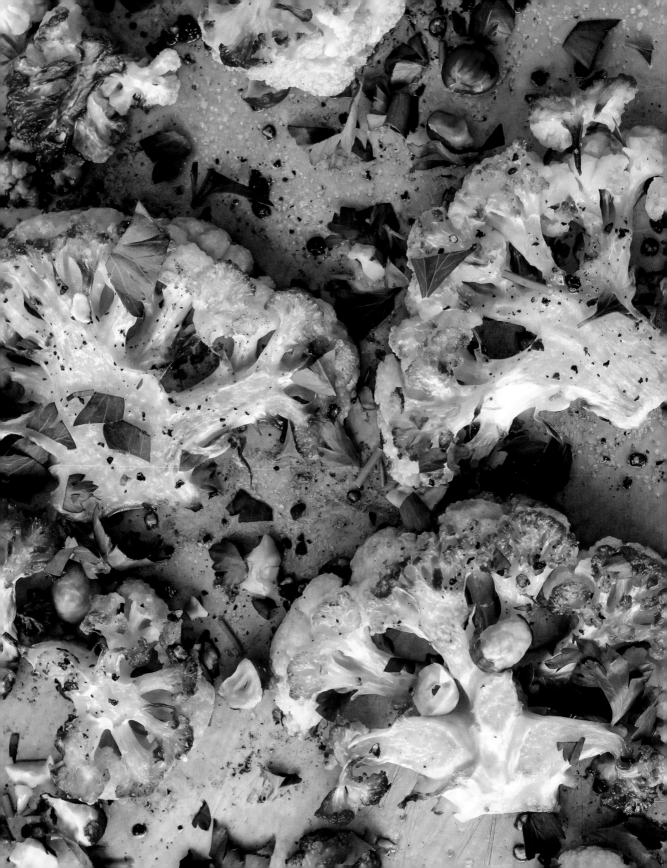

CHAPTER 10

Keto-Green Plant-Based Detox Recipes

To view videos of the preparation of some of the recipes in this plan, go to dranna.com/menupause-extras.

*These recipes can be used in other plans as well. See the recipe pages for more information.

Grain-Free Granola MAKES 9 (½-CUP) SERVINGS

Vegetable oil cooking spray

1 cup unsalted hulled sunflower seeds

1 cup unsalted hulled pumpkin seeds

½ cup hemp seeds

½ cup sesame seeds

1 cup sliced almonds

1 cup pecan pieces

¾ cup unsweetened coconut flakes

2 tablespoons Mighty Maca Plus, or 1 tablespoon maca root powder

½ cup coconut oil, melted

1 tablespoon vanilla extract

2 tablespoons ground cinnamon

2 teaspoons ground nutmeg

½ teaspoon sea salt

½ cup dried cherries

I have always loved traditional granola, but it is so high in sugar and carbs, and it definitely is not keto friendly. But here's some great news: you can make a grain-free, keto granola with nuts and seeds as the base, and it tastes even better than its namesake. Also, nuts and seeds are excellent for balancing hormones, easing menopause symptoms, and increasing dietary fiber.

Preheat the oven to 350°F. Coat a baking sheet with cooking spray.

In a large bowl, mix the seeds, nuts, coconut flakes, and maca powder. In a small bowl, mix the coconut oil, vanilla, cinnamon, nutmeg, and salt. Add to the seed/nut mixture, and using your hands, mix well, making sure that the ingredients are well coated with oil.

Spread the mixture evenly on the prepared baking sheet and bake for 10 minutes. Stir the mixture to ensure even baking and return the baking sheet to the oven for another 10 minutes.

Stir in the cherries and bake for a final 5 minutes, watching carefully to make sure nothing burns.

Let the mixture cool on the baking sheet, then transfer to a lidded container and store in the refrigerator.

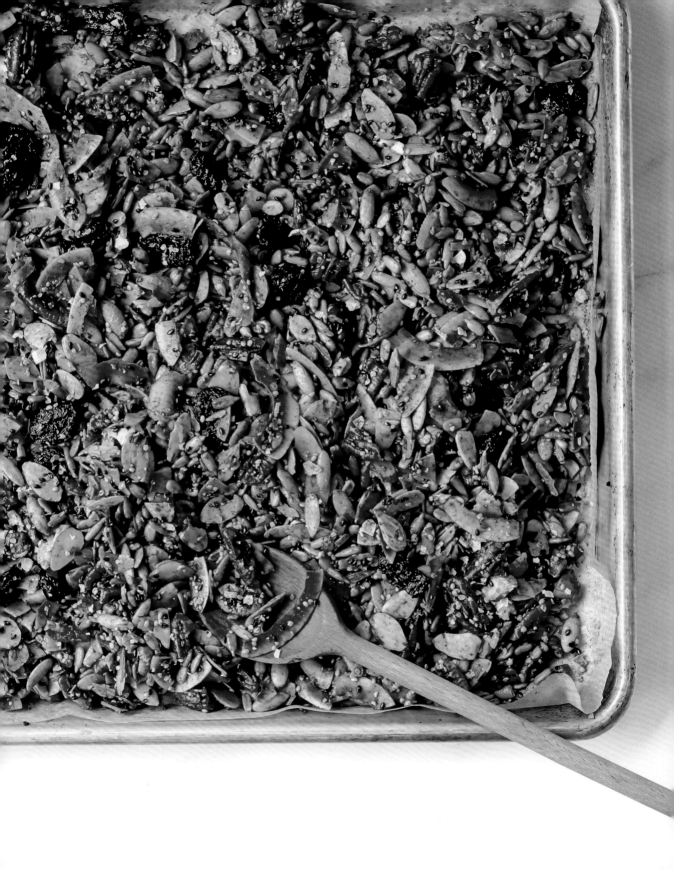

Garden Salad in a Shake

MAKES 1 SERVING

1½ cups unsweetened coconut milk

2 tablespoons chilled cream from full-fat coconut milk (skimmed off top of refrigerated can)

¾ cup frozen strawberries

Handful of fresh spinach

1 scoop Dr. Anna's Keto-Green Shake or Dr. Anna's Keto-Alkaline Protein Shake (see Note)

2 scoops Mighty Maca Plus, or 1 teaspoon maca root powder

If you want a great green smoothie with a little sweetness, this is it. This shake is as healthy as a big green salad but makes a quick on-the-go breakfast. The spinach pumps up the alkalinizing benefits of the smoothie.

Place the coconut milk, coconut cream, strawberries, spinach, protein powder, and maca in a blender, and blend until smooth. A trick I learned to coax my daughter into enjoying shakes when she was little was to add a small slice of beet. It turns the shake into a beautiful rosy red color.

NOTE: Or, substitute a good protein powder formulated with a vegan protein such as pea or rice protein and containing less than 3 grams of sugar (per serving) and less than 10 grams of carbohydrate (per serving).

Mexican Mushrooms MAKES 2 SERVINGS

1 (12-ounce) package button mushrooms, stems removed

⅓ cup extra-virgin olive oil

⅓ cup distilled white vinegar

2 garlic cloves, minced

1 teaspoon red pepper flakes

½ teaspoon dried Mexican oregano

½ teaspoon sea salt

1 large onion, thinly sliced and separated into rings

Lettuce leaves

If you're looking for vegan dishes or just some delicious ways to cook veggies, these marinated mushrooms are a tasty option. Mushrooms are so meaty-tasting and they pair well with other vegetables. They are also one of the few plant foods rich in hormone-balancing vitamin D.

Place oil, vinegar, garlic, red pepper flakes, oregano, and salt in a small saucepan. Add enough water to fill halfway. Bring to a boil, then add the onion rings. Cook over medium heat until the onion is tender.

Place the mushrooms in a medium bowl and pour the onion mixture over them. Let them sit for 2 hours at room temperature, stirring frequently, then drain and chill until ready to serve.

Spread the lettuce leaves on serving plates and scatter the mushrooms over. Enjoy.

NOTE: This recipe can also be used on the Keto-Green Extreme Plan (without the red pepper flakes) and Carbohydrate Modification Plan as a side dish.

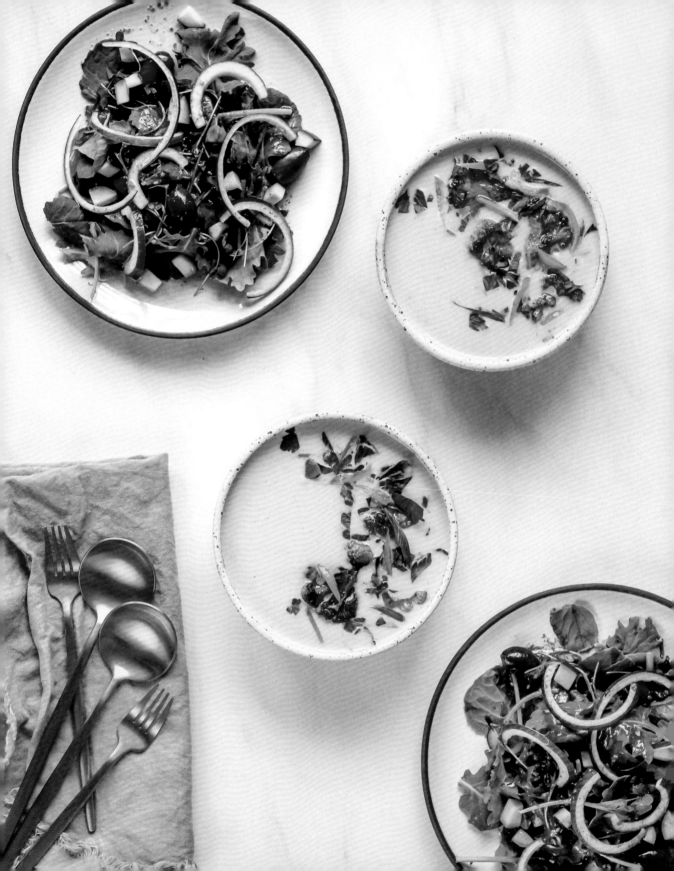

Tahini Cauliflower Soup

MAKES 4 SERVINGS

For the soup

- 2 tablespoons extra-virgin olive oil
- 1 medium onion, chopped
- 6 garlic cloves, chopped
- 1 small head cauliflower, cored and cut into florets (see Note)
- 1 teaspoon ground cumin
- ½ teaspoon ground coriander
- ½ teaspoon paprika
- Sea salt and black pepper
- 4 cups vegetable broth
- ¼ cup tahini
- Juice of 1 lemon
- Crispy Cauliflower Florets (optional; recipe follows)
- Minced preserved lemon (optional)
- Chopped fresh parsley

NOTE: This soup pairs well with the Greek Keto-Green Salad (page 137).

Tahini is a butter-like paste made from toasted and ground sesame seeds. Considered a staple of Mediterranean cuisine, it is also used in Asian, Middle Eastern, and African dishes. Most often associated with hummus, tahini is versatile and can be used to flavor soups, as done here. A lesser-known fact about tahini is that it is rich in phytoestrogens, meaning that it can be beneficial for transitioning through menopause. Not only that, but it also helps maintain hormonal balance and controls and reduces hormonal fluctuations. This soup can be made on the stovetop or in a slow cooker.

Stovetop Directions

Heat the olive oil in a large pot over medium-high heat. When the oil is hot, add the onion and garlic and cook for 2 to 3 minutes, until the onion softens and becomes translucent. Add the cauliflower, cumin, coriander, paprika, and a pinch each of salt and pepper. Toss to coat well, then add the broth.

Bring to a boil, then reduce the heat to medium-low, cover the pot, and cook for 25 to 30 minutes, until the cauliflower is fork-tender.

Transfer the cauliflower mixture to a blender, add the tahini and lemon juice, and blend until smooth. Taste and adjust with salt and pepper, if necessary. Top with

(recipe continues)

NOTE: If making the crispy cauliflower, reserve about ½ cup of florets; otherwise, use entire batch for the soup.

NOTE: This recipe can also be used on the Carbohydrate Modification Plan. Feel free to add a carbohydrate as a side dish.

the crispy cauliflower, if desired. Sprinkle with the preserved lemon and the parsley, then serve.

Slow Cooker Directions

Combine the olive oil, onion, garlic, cauliflower, cumin, coriander, paprika, salt and pepper, and broth in a slow cooker. Cover and cook on high for 3 to 4 hours, until the cauliflower is fork-tender.

Transfer the mix to a blender, add the tahini and lemon juice, and blend until smooth. Taste and adjust salt and pepper, if necessary. Top with the crispy cauliflower, if desired. Sprinkle the soup with the preserved lemon and parsley garnish and serve.

Crispy Cauliflower Florets

MAKES ABOUT ½ CUP

1 to 2 teaspoons extra-virgin olive oil

½ cup small cauliflower florets

Sea salt and black pepper

Pinch of ground cumin

Pinch of ground coriander

Pinch of paprika

Ground nutmeg, for garnish (optional)

While the soup cooks, you can prepare the crispy cauliflower garnish. Heat the olive oil in a small skillet over medium-high heat. When the oil is hot, add the cauliflower and season with salt and pepper and the cumin, coriander, and paprika. Cook, stirring occasionally, for about 8 minutes, until the cauliflower is tender and the edges turn golden brown. When ready to scatter atop the soup, dust with the nutmeg, if desired.

Tangle of Greens

MAKES 2 SERVINGS

The more greens you eat when going Keto-Green, the more alkaline your body can become. An alkaline body is the healthiest state you can achieve. It is good for your bones, joints, brain, muscles—and helps with weight loss, too.

2 tablespoons extra-virgin olive oil

1 tablespoon minced shallot

1 teaspoon minced garlic

1½ cups fresh baby spinach

1 cup arugula

Sea salt and black pepper

Heat the olive oil in a large skillet over medium-high heat. Add the shallot and garlic and sauté for 1 minute. Add the spinach and arugula and sauté until the greens have wilted, about 3 minutes. Season to taste with salt and pepper and serve.

NOTE: This recipe can also be used on the Keto-Green Extreme Plan (without the black pepper) and Carbohydrate Modification Plan as a side dish.

Arabic Garden Salad

MAKES 2 SERVINGS

Here is another favorite from my heritage. Enjoy the variety of flavors and textures it offers, with its mingling of veggies with mint, which is good for easing tummy troubles.

3 ripe medium tomatoes, chopped

1 large cucumber, chopped

½ head Romaine lettuce, chopped

1 small onion, chopped

1 teaspoon dried mint, or 1 tablespoon fresh

2 tablespoons extra-virgin olive oil

Juice of 1 lemon

Sea salt

Combine all the ingredients in a bowl. Toss well, then serve.

NOTE: This recipe can also be used on the Carbohydrate Modification Plan as a side dish.

Tomato Salad

MAKES 2 SERVINGS

3 ripe medium tomatoes

1 green bell pepper

½ bunch scallions
(about 3)

1 medium cucumber

4 red radishes, trimmed
and sliced

½ bunch fresh parsley

1 tablespoon chopped
fresh mint,
or 1 teaspoon dried

1 garlic clove, crushed

¼ cup extra-virgin olive
oil

Juice of 2 lemons

Sea salt and black
pepper

Here's a side dish that's as colorful as it is tasty. Fresh tomatoes combine with other veggies and herbs to create a simple and refreshing salad full of flavor. Botanically a fruit, tomatoes are thought of mostly as a vegetable. They are high in lycopene, which has been studied for its protective properties when it comes to breast and other cancers.

Wash and coarsely chop the tomatoes, green pepper, scallions, and cucumber and add to a medium bowl. Add the radishes, parsley, mint, garlic, olive oil, and lemon juice. Toss and then let marinate for 30 minutes.

When ready to serve, season with salt and pepper.

NOTE: This recipe can also be used on the Carbohydrate Modification Plan as a side dish.

Keto-Green Hummus

MAKES 2 TO 4 SERVINGS

1 (14-ounce) can chickpeas, drained and rinsed

1 cup baby spinach leaves

3 tablespoons tahini

Juice of 1 lemon

2 garlic cloves

¼ cup extra-virgin olive oil

2 tablespoons filtered water

1 teaspoon sea salt, or more as needed

½ teaspoon ground cumin

I love my Keto-Green smoothies, so I started thinking, *Why not a Keto-Green hummus?* So, I whipped one up, adding spinach to a basic hummus recipe. What a delicious and nutrition boost to a classic dip! Serve this with raw veggies, such as cucumber slices, zucchini sticks, baby carrots, or celery ribs. Remember, too, that chickpeas have a long list of menopause-easing benefits. For example, they support digestive health and build denser bones.

Place the chickpeas in a food processor or blender and add the remaining ingredients. Blend until smooth and creamy. Adjust the seasoning with more salt, if needed. Serve as a dip.

NOTE: This recipe can also be used on the Carbohydrate Modification Plan.

Spicy Gazpacho MAKES 2 SERVINGS

1 pound ripe tomatoes (preferably Roma or plum), halved and seeded

½ small cucumber, peeled and seeded

½ green bell pepper, cored and seeded

¼ cup chopped red onion

1 small garlic clove

1½ tablespoons extra-virgin olive oil

1 tablespoon sherry vinegar

½ teaspoon sea salt

¼ teaspoon black pepper

¼ teaspoon ground cumin

Legend has it that Christopher Columbus took a soup made with bread bits, olive oil, garlic, water, and a few vegetables with him on his voyages from Spain. After he brought back tomatoes, cucumbers, and various peppers from the New World, these vegetables were put into his traveling soup. That soup has evolved to its present state, a blend of vegetables with a tomato base. Gazpacho is widely eaten in Spain and Portugal, particularly during hot summers, when it is served cold. This mixture of so many vegetables brings digestive health, heart health, and other benefits to the table.

Place the tomatoes, cucumber, bell pepper, red onion, garlic, olive oil, and vinegar in a blender or food processor. Puree for 1 minute, until fairly smooth but with some small chunks remaining. Taste and season with the salt, pepper, and cumin.

Transfer to a sealed container and refrigerate for 3 to 4 hours, or until completely chilled.

Serve cold.

NOTE: This recipe can also be used on the Carbohydrate Modification Plan. Feel free to add a carbohydrate as a side dish.

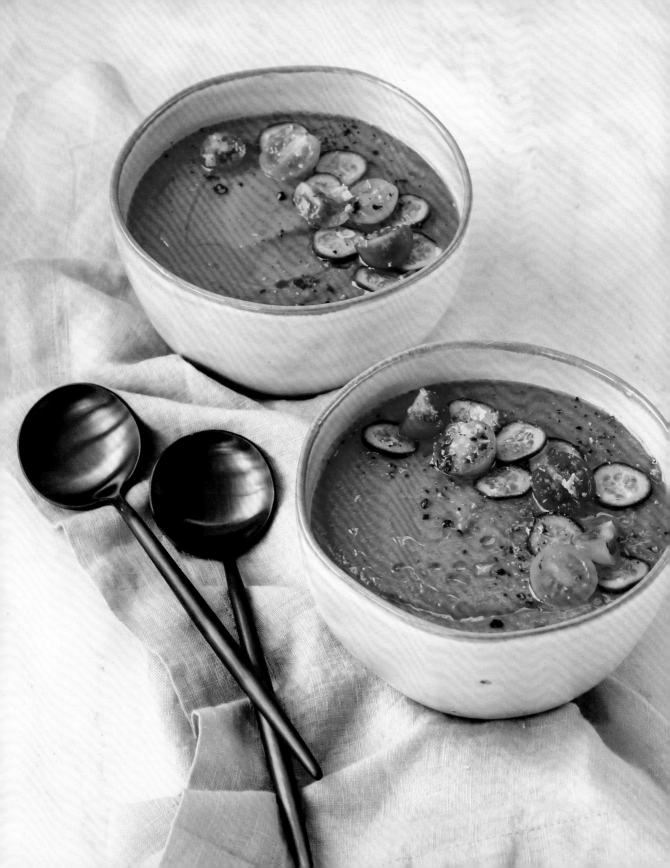

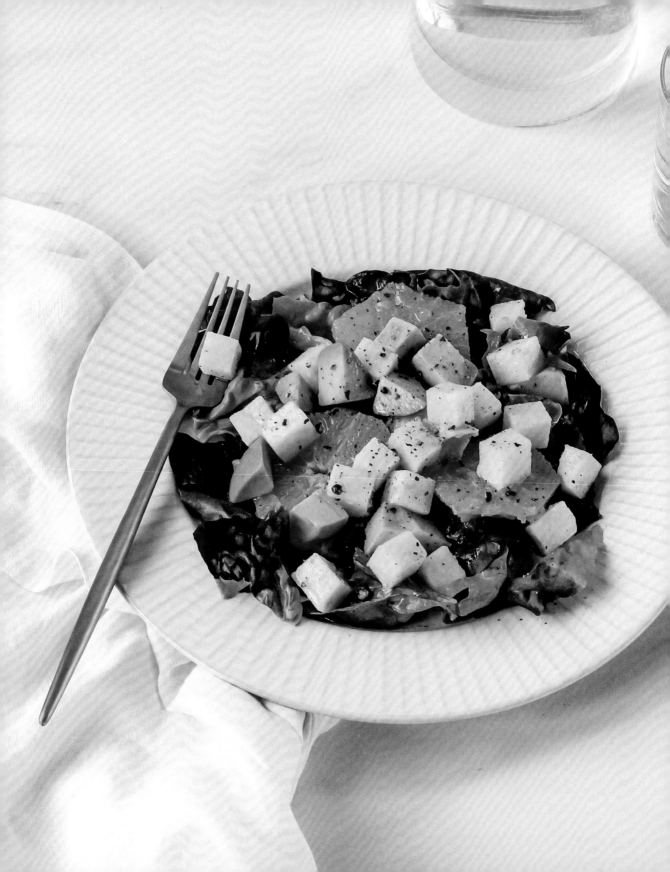

Jicama Salad   MAKES 2 SERVINGS

¼ cup minced fresh cilantro

2 tablespoons fresh lime juice

2 tablespoons white wine vinegar

2 tablespoons extra-virgin olive oil

½ teaspoon sea salt

¼ teaspoon black pepper

3 oranges, peeled and cut into ¼-inch-thick slices

1 avocado, cut into ½-inch cubes

1 small jicama, peeled and cut into ½-inch cubes

Red lettuce leaves

Jicama is a globe-shaped root vegetable similar to a turnip and with lots of health benefits. For one thing, it is low in carbs, so it fits in perfectly with the Keto-Green crowd of foods. Plus, jicama provides a satisfying crunch.

In a medium bowl, combine the cilantro, lime juice, vinegar, olive oil, and salt and pepper. Whisk together until well combined. Add the oranges, avocado, and jicama and allow to marinate in the refrigerator for 30 minutes.

Arrange the lettuce on plates. Drain the jicama mixture and place on the lettuce. Serve.

NOTE: This recipe can also be used on the Carbohydrate Modification Plan as a side dish.

Red Lentil and Squash Soup

MAKES 2 SERVINGS

1 butternut squash, peeled, seeded, and cut into 1-inch pieces

3 to 4 tablespoons extra-virgin olive oil

1 medium onion, finely chopped

2 garlic cloves, crushed

¾ teaspoon cumin seeds

¾ teaspoon coriander seeds

½ teaspoon ground cinnamon

¾ cup red lentils, rinsed

3 cups vegetable broth

Sea salt and black pepper

2 tablespoons za'atar blend or dried thyme

Chopped fresh parsley or cilantro

My mom loved making this soup in the winter. The main ingredient she used was protein-packed lentils, as I've used here. Her version included rice, but I wanted to downsize the carbs a bit, so I use squash instead. Butternut squash is an antioxidant-rich food. In particular, it gets its orange color from a group of antioxidants that is important for memory and mental functioning, called carotenoids. You'll love this hearty soup; it's such a grounding, warming meal, especially when you feel anxious or stressed.

Preheat the oven to 400°F.

Arrange the butternut squash chunks on a baking sheet and drizzle them with some of the olive oil. Toss the chunks so they are evenly coated with the oil, then roast for 20 to 30 minutes, until tender.

Heat 3 tablespoons of the olive oil in a large saucepan over medium-high heat. Add the onion and sauté for 5 minutes over medium heat, until translucent. Add the garlic, reduce the heat to low, and cook for another few minutes, until soft.

Place the cumin and coriander seeds in a dry skillet over low heat, and stir for about 1 minute to toast them. Crush the seeds in a mortar and pestle or grind them in a spice grinder. Add the ground seeds, along with the cinnamon, to the saucepan with the onion. Stir together for a few minutes on low, then remove from heat.

Place the lentils in a large pot over medium heat and

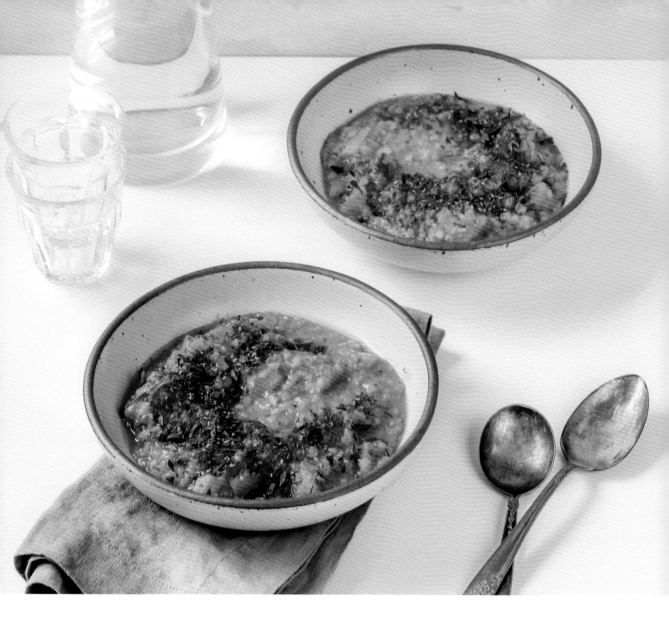

add the broth. Cook for 20 to 25 minutes, until tender. Add the onion-spice mixture and the squash, stirring to blend and heat through. Season to taste with salt and pepper.

Serve the soup with the za'atar and parsley sprinkled on top.

NOTE: This recipe can also be used on the Carbohydrate Modification Plan.

Golden Cabbage Chickpea Soup

MAKES 2 SERVINGS

1 tablespoon extra-virgin olive oil

1 medium onion, chopped

4 garlic cloves, chopped

1 small head green cabbage, cored and chopped

2 celery stalks, chopped

1 large carrot, chopped

Sea salt and black pepper

1 cup drained and rinsed canned chickpeas

Juice of 1 lemon

4 to 6 cups vegetable broth

½ teaspoon ground turmeric

½ teaspoon ground cumin

½ teaspoon ground coriander

¼ teaspoon cayenne

Lemon wedges (optional)

Chopped fresh parsley (optional)

Here's a delicious twist on cabbage soup: add chickpeas. Also called garbanzo beans, these legumes have a buttery, nutty flavor and a creamy texture—perfect as a soup ingredient. Plus, they are a great source of fiber and plant-based protein, as well as having a load of nutrients, like folate and iron. A meal in itself, this soup is easily made on the stovetop or in a slow cooker.

Stovetop Directions

Heat the olive oil in a large pot over medium-high heat. Add the onion and garlic and cook for 2 to 3 minutes, until the onion softens and becomes translucent. Add the cabbage, celery, and carrot. Season with salt and pepper and cook for another 3 minutes, then add the chickpeas and lemon juice.

Start adding the broth, beginning with 4 cups and continuing until all the vegetables are covered.

Adjust the salt and pepper as needed and add the turmeric, cumin, coriander, and cayenne. Bring to a boil, then reduce the heat to medium-low, cover the pot, and cook for 25 to 30 minutes, until the vegetables are tender.

Serve the soup with the lemon wedges and chopped parsley, if desired.

Slow Cooker Directions

In a slow cooker, combine the olive oil, onion, garlic, cabbage, celery, carrot, chickpeas, and lemon juice. Add enough broth to cover the vegetables, Then add the salt, pepper, turmeric, cumin, coriander, and cayenne. Cover the cooker and set to cook on high for 3 to 4 hours. When ready to serve, taste and adjust the salt and pepper as needed, then serve with the lemon wedges and chopped parsley, if desired.

NOTE: This recipe can also be used on the Carbohydrate Modification Plan. Feel free to add a carbohydrate as a side dish.

Dr. Anna's Keto-Green Tabbouleh

MAKES 2 SERVINGS

2 cups broccoli sprouts

1 cup chopped cucumber

¾ cup chopped cherry tomatoes

4 scallions (white and green parts), thinly sliced

⅓ cup chopped fresh mint

2 cups packed chopped fresh parsley

For the dressing

4 garlic cloves, mashed

Juice of 1 lemon, or more as needed

½ teaspoon sea salt, or more as needed

¼ to ½ cup extra-virgin olive oil

I grew up eating a lot of tabbouleh, and I love this healthful salad. Normally, tabbouleh features high-carb bulgur wheat as its main ingredient. Of course, I tinkered with it a bit to downsize the carbs by swapping in broccoli sprouts for the wheat, making it right for this plan. Nonetheless, it's still absolutely delicious and one of my go-to comfort foods. One of its noteworthy ingredients is parsley, a natural diuretic and anti-inflammatory food.

Place the sprouts in a large bowl. Add the cucumber, tomatoes, scallions, mint, and parsley. Mix well.

Whisk together the dressing ingredients. Pour the dressing over the vegetable mixture and toss to coat. Add more salt and lemon juice to the dressing, if desired. Serve the salad immediately or refrigerate to let the flavors meld. It tastes even better the second day, so consider doubling the recipe.

NOTE: This recipe can also be used on the Carbohydrate Modification Plan as a side dish.

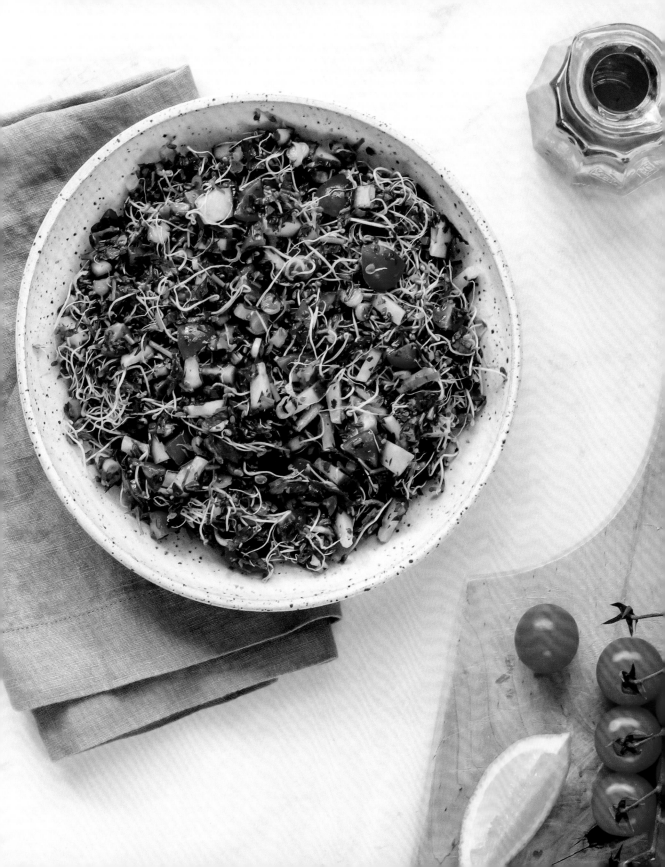

Kale and Tempeh Tacos   MAKES 2 SERVINGS

1 tablespoon extra-virgin olive oil

1 small onion, chopped

2 garlic cloves, chopped

4 ounces tempeh, cubed

½ teaspoon sea salt, or more as needed

½ teaspoon black pepper, or more as needed

½ teaspoon ground cumin

½ teaspoon chili powder

¼ teaspoon paprika

¼ teaspoon cayenne

¼ cup vegetable broth

2 cups stemmed and chopped fresh kale

4 to 6 large green cabbage leaves, dipped for 30 seconds into hot water to soften

½ avocado, sliced

1 radish, sliced

¼ cup chopped fresh cilantro

½ lime, cut into wedges

In this yummy recipe, cabbage leaves substitute for the tortillas and are filled with a mixture of protein-packed tempeh, veggies, and lots of great spices, making these low-carb, super-delicious "tacos." Compounds in tempeh called isoflavones are known to serve as a natural remedy for menopausal relief.

Heat the olive oil in a large skillet over medium-high heat. Add the onion, garlic, and tempeh and cook for 2 to 3 minutes, until the onion softens and becomes translucent.

Add the salt, pepper, cumin, chili powder, paprika, and cayenne, stir, then add the broth and kale. Stir to combine and cook until the broth thickens and reduces by at least one-half. Taste and adjust the salt and pepper as needed.

Spread the cabbage leaves open on a large plate. Spoon the kale mixture into the center of the leaves. Add some of the avocado, radish slices, and cilantro, then fold in the sides like a taco. Serve with lime wedges.

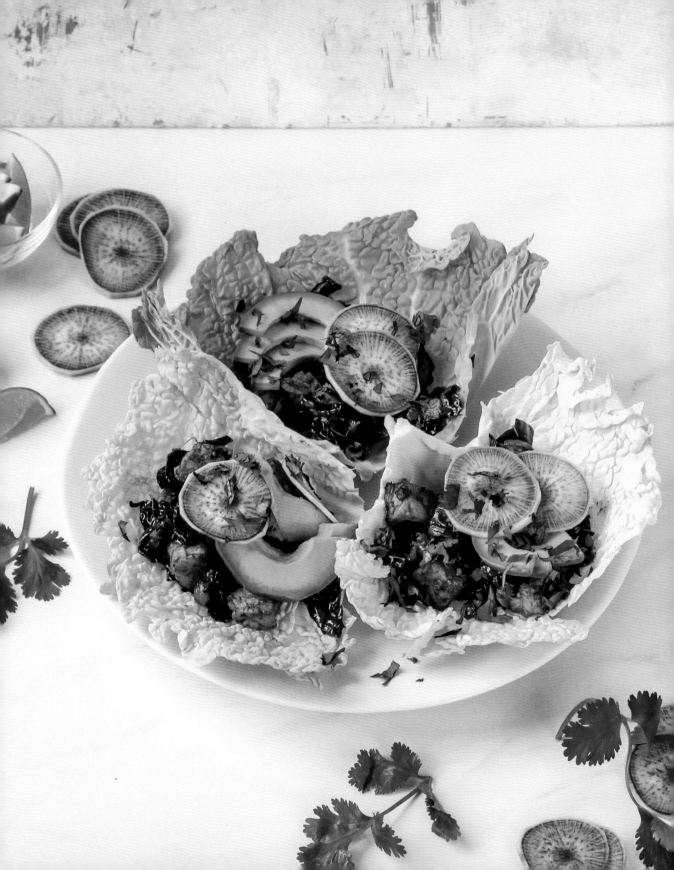

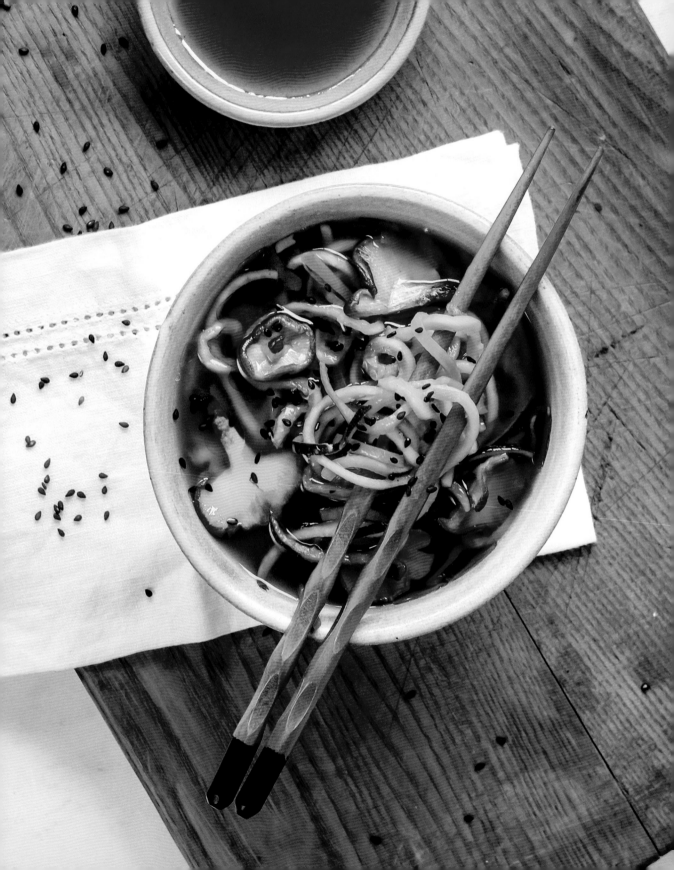

Miso-Ginger Zoodle Ramen

MAKES 2 SERVINGS

3 tablespoons extra-virgin olive oil (2 tablespoons for stovetop cooking)

1 medium onion, halved and sliced

4 garlic cloves, chopped

¼ cup shredded carrot

1 tablespoon grated fresh ginger

1 tablespoon white miso paste

1 tablespoon coconut aminos

3½ cups vegetable broth

Sea salt and black pepper

1½ cups chopped shiitake mushrooms

1 large zucchini, spiralized or sliced paper-thin

2 cups chopped mustard greens or bok choy or spinach

Toasted sesame oil (optional)

White sesame seeds (optional)

This dish begins with a super-savory combination of onion, garlic, ginger, carrot, and miso (which is essential for the salty flavor that ramen is known for). Then, I add the spiralized zucchini (zoodles), which are the perfect low-carb swap for the traditional ramen noodles. Other veggies, like mushrooms and mustard greens, add additional healing power. Of course, to make this you will need a spiralizer; as an alternative, you can slice the zucchini on a mandoline slicer. The dish can be made on the stovetop or in a slow cooker.

Stovetop Directions

Heat 2 tablespoons of the olive oil in a large pot over medium-high heat. Add the onion, garlic, and carrot and cook for 2 to 3 minutes, until the onion softens and becomes translucent. Add the ginger and miso, stir, and cook for another 2 minutes. Add the coconut aminos and broth, then season with salt and pepper. Bring to a boil, then reduce the heat to medium-low and simmer for 20 minutes.

While the miso broth simmers, heat the remaining tablespoon olive oil in a medium skillet over medium-high heat. Add the mushrooms, season with salt and pepper, and sauté for 8 to 10 minutes, until the mushrooms become tender.

Transfer the mushrooms to the miso broth. Add the zucchini and greens, cover the pot, and cook for another 5 to 10 minutes, until the zoodles are tender and the greens are wilted.

(recipe continues)

Serve, if desired, with a small drizzle of the sesame oil and pinch of sesame seeds on top.

Slow Cooker Directions

In a slow cooker, combine the onion, garlic, carrot, ginger, miso, coconut aminos, and broth. Stir to combine, season with salt and pepper, cover, and set to cook on high for 2 to 3 hours.

Twenty minutes before you plan to serve, heat 1 tablespoon olive oil in a medium skillet over medium-high heat. Add the mushrooms, season with salt and pepper, and sauté for 8 to 10 minutes, until the mushrooms become tender.

Transfer the mushrooms, zucchini, and greens to the slow cooker. Cover and cook for another 5 to 10 minutes, until the zoodles are tender and the greens are wilted.

Serve, if desired, with a small drizzle of the sesame oil and a pinch of the sesame seeds on top.

Comforting Spinach and Chickpeas MAKES 3 SERVINGS

4 tablespoons extra-virgin olive oil

½ medium onion, finely chopped

½ teaspoon cumin seeds

½ teaspoon coriander seeds

2 garlic cloves, crushed

¼ teaspoon ground allspice

¼ teaspoon ground nutmeg

½ teaspoon black pepper

1 teaspoon sea salt

1 (14-ounce) can chickpeas, drained and rinsed

1 cup vegetable broth

1 (16-ounce) bag fresh spinach, roughly chopped

2 tablespoons fresh lemon juice

Here's an easy-to-fix plant-based entree that combines two of my favorite vegetables—spinach and chickpeas—with a number of Mediterranean spices. It is truly a comforting meal for cold nights, or whenever you just need to whip up something quickly. Coriander and cumin effectively support healthy digestion.

Heat 2 tablespoons of the olive oil in a large saucepan over a medium heat. Add the onion and sauté for 10 minutes, until tender.

Place the cumin and coriander seeds in a dry skillet over low heat and toast for a minute or so. Grind the seeds in a mortar and pestle or a spice grinder, then add to the saucepan along with the garlic, allspice, nutmeg, and ½ teaspoon pepper. Sauté for a few minutes, then add the chickpeas and broth. Cover and simmer for 15 minutes, until everything is heated though.

Add the spinach, lemon juice, 1 teaspoon salt, and the remaining 2 tablespoons olive oil. Cook for 5 to 10 minutes, then serve.

NOTE: This recipe can also be used on the Carbohydrate Modification Plan as a side dish.

Mushroom and Kale Stew MAKES 4 SERVINGS

2 tablespoons extra-virgin olive oil

2 small shallots, chopped

4 garlic cloves, chopped

8 ounces fresh shiitake or cremini mushrooms, sliced

4 ounces fresh wild mushrooms (chanterelle, oyster, etc.), sliced

Sea salt and black pepper

1 teaspoon chopped fresh thyme

¼ teaspoon red pepper flakes

3 cups vegetable broth

2 cups stemmed and chopped Tuscan kale

I can't get enough of mushrooms, because of their meaty taste and the benefits they offer to hormonal health, so I use them here as the base for a savory stew. Serve this to your omnivore friends, and they won't know that it doesn't have meat in it.

Heat 1 tablespoon of the olive oil in a large pot over medium-high heat. Add the shallots and garlic and cook for 3 to 4 minutes, until shallots are translucent and garlic is golden brown. Use a slotted spoon to remove the shallots and garlic.

Add the remaining tablespoons of oil to the pot. When hot, add the mushrooms and cook, stirring, for 2 minutes. Season with salt and pepper, thyme, and red pepper flakes, and cook for another 2 minutes.

Add the shallots and garlic back to the pot. Add the broth and bring to a boil, then reduce the heat to medium-low and simmer for 20 minutes. Five minutes before serving, stir in the kale and cook about 5 minutes, until fully wilted. Adjust the salt and pepper as needed and serve.

NOTE: This recipe can also be used on the Keto-Green Extreme Plan (without the black pepper and the red pepper flakes) and the Carbohydrate Modification Plan as a side dish.

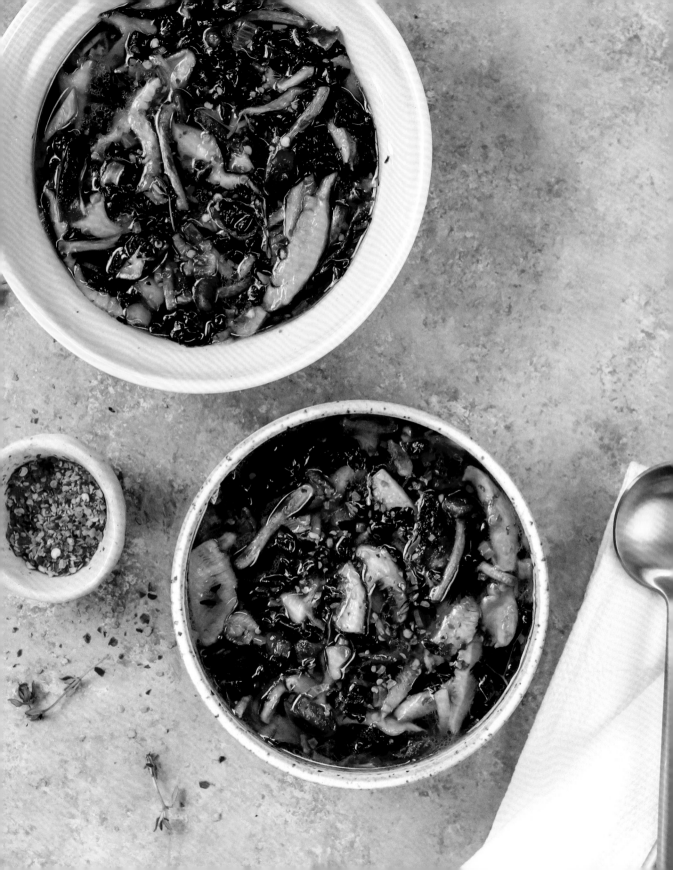

Roasted Cauliflower Steaks

MAKES 2 SERVINGS

1 large head of cauliflower, cored and cut lengthwise into 4 (1-inch-thick) slices

Extra-virgin olive oil

Sea salt and black pepper

1 tablespoon pili nuts or hazelnuts

2 tablespoons chopped fresh parsley

Sure, I love a juicy ribeye steak every now and then, but I make it a practice to abstain from animal foods several times a year. When I do this, I always make these "steaks." They're so yummy, especially with an alkalinizing green salad on the side. Pili nuts are a low-carb, buttery-tasting nut used often in Asian dishes.

Preheat the oven to 425°F.

Arrange the cauliflower slices on a baking sheet in a single layer. Drizzle with the olive oil and season with salt and pepper on both sides. Bake 20 to 25 minutes, until golden brown, turning over after the first 10 minutes.

Sprinkle the nuts over the cauliflower and continue to bake for 5 more minutes.

Transfer the "steaks" to a platter to serve and top with the parsley.

NOTE: This recipe can also be used on the Carbohydrate Modification Plan as a side dish.

Stovetop Ratatouille

MAKES 2 SERVINGS

4 tablespoons extra-virgin olive oil

1 medium onion, coarsely chopped

1 teaspoon minced garlic

1 red bell pepper, cored and cut into 1-inch pieces

1 medium eggplant, cut into 1-inch cubes

2 medium zucchini, cut in half lengthwise and then crosswise into ¼-inch slices

½ cup sliced fresh mushrooms

1 (28-ounce) can diced tomatoes, drained

Sea salt and black pepper

As a poor medical student, I had to squeeze my food pennies. One of the most economical ways to do that was to cook a huge batch of this mouthwatering ratatouille and eat it throughout the week. Although my mom called it "poor man's stew," it's super-rich in healthy brain food and has lots of hormone-balancing nutrients.

Heat the olive oil in a large saucepan. Add the onion, garlic, and bell pepper. Sauté for about 5 minutes, until the vegetables are tender.

Add the eggplant, zucchini, and mushrooms and continue to cook for about 8 minutes, stirring often. Stir in the tomatoes and season with salt and pepper. Lower the heat to a simmer and cook for another 20 to 30 minutes, stirring occasionally. Serve at once or transfer to airtight containers and refrigerate.

NOTE: This recipe can also be used on the Carbohydrate Modification Plan as a side dish in a smaller portion.

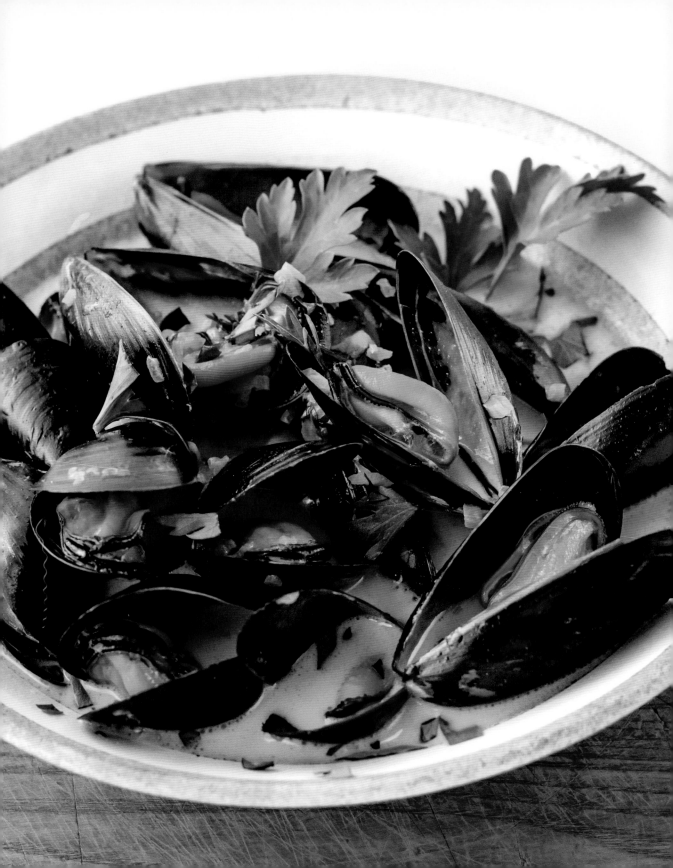

CHAPTER 11

The Carbohydrate Pause Recipes

To view videos of some of the recipes in this plan, go to dranna.com/menupause-extras.

* These recipes can be used in other plans as well. See the recipe pages for more information.

Spicy Diablo Eggs   MAKES 2 SERVINGS

2 large eggs, hard-boiled

¼ avocado, diced

1 strip (no-sugar) bacon, cooked until crisp and chopped

1 teaspoon fresh lime juice

¼ teaspoon habanero flakes (optional)

¼ teaspoon minced garlic

Pinch of cayenne

Pinch of sea salt

4 slices jalapeño pepper (optional)

I have loved deviled eggs all my life. They bring back memories of family celebrations, picnics, and holidays. There are so many ways to make them, too. In this recipe, I've spiced them up a bit and added bacon for a truly satisfying, high-protein meal. Eggs are rich in vitamin D and full of iron, both nutrients that women often lack. They are also a great protein source for menopausal women and have been shown to reduce the chances of heart disease and obesity.

Peel the eggs, then cut in half lengthwise. Remove the yolks and place in a small bowl.

Add the avocado, two-thirds of the bacon bits, the lime juice, habanero (if using), garlic, cayenne, and salt. Mash the egg yolks and avocado until smooth.

Spoon the mixture into the egg whites, smoothing the tops a bit. Place a jalapeño slice on each (if using) and serve.

NOTE: This recipe can also be used on the Carbohydrate Modification Plan as a breakfast entree.

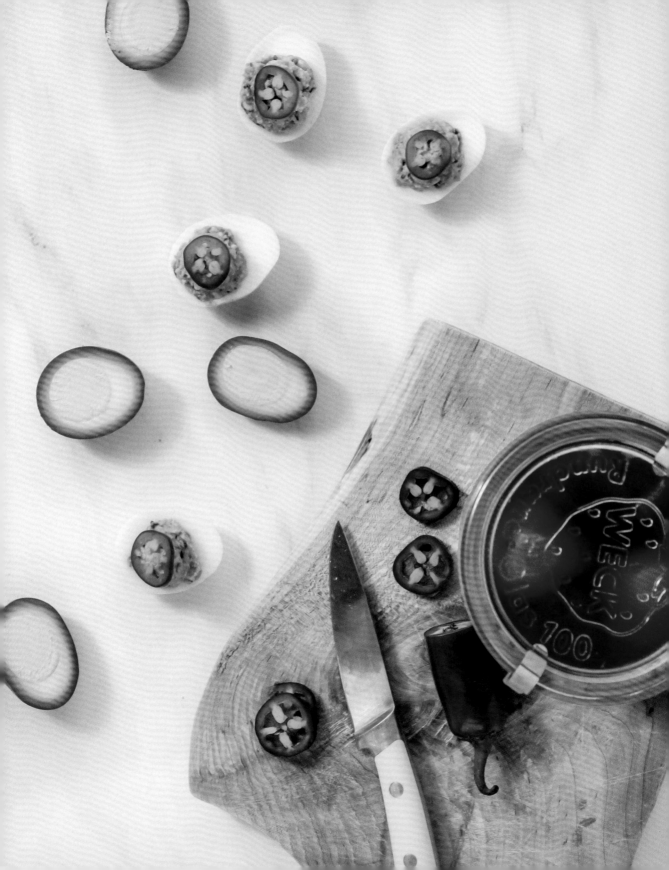

Pickled Beet Eggs MAKES 2 TO 3 SERVINGS

6 large eggs, hard-boiled

1 (14-ounce) can sliced beets, or 1 cup cooked, peeled, and sliced fresh beets

¼ cup distilled white vinegar

Filtered water

NOTE: This recipe can also be used on the Carbohydrate Modification Plan as a breakfast entree.

Did you know that you can pickle eggs? Absolutely—and they are spectacular in flavor. Plus, they make a unique breakfast dish, if you want to enjoy a different twist on your morning eggs. I like to pickle mine with beets, one of the healthiest veggies on the planet. You must try these; you won't be disappointed.

Peel the eggs and place in a large glass jar that has a well-fitting lid. Spoon the beets and any canning liquid over the eggs, then add the vinegar. Top off with filtered water to within ½-inch headspace, covering the eggs and beets. Stir with a knife to settle the ingredients and release any air bubbles.

Place a layer of plastic wrap on top of the jar, then screw on the lid. Refrigerate for at least 24 hours, and up to 48 hours for the best results.

Variations: Try the following for a different twist on pickled eggs, but be sure to dissolve any spices before adding the eggs to the jar.

- Add the brine from a jar of dill pickles
- Include a garlic clove or sliced small onion
- Add a sliced jalapeño pepper
- Stir in some whole cloves or a piece of cinnamon stick for spicy sweetness
- Stir in a pinch of cayenne or sprinkle in some red pepper flakes for hotness
- Add prepared pickling spice (available in the spice section of the grocery store) to the liquid
- Use apple cider vinegar instead of white vinegar

Scotch Eggs

MAKES 2 SERVINGS

4 large eggs, hard-boiled

8 ounces ground pork sausage

Like many recipes, this one has a long history. Scotch eggs are said to have been introduced by Fortnum & Mason, a luxury London department store, in the 18th century, and were served as a shoppers' snack. They were popular back then, without the now-common breadcrumb layer, even as they are today. Scotch eggs make the perfect high-protein, no-carb meal with only the original two ingredients, as prepared here for the Carbohydrate Pause. It's a great way to start the day.

Preheat the oven to 350°F. Line a baking sheet with parchment paper.

Peel the eggs. Divide the sausage into 4 equal portions and form each into a thin round patty.

Put the sausage rounds on a work surface. Place an egg in the center of each round, then pick up the meat and egg in the palm of your hand. With your other hand, shape and mold the meat around the egg. Smooth the outside of the ovals so that the egg is covered completely with the sausage.

Place the eggs on the prepared baking sheet and bake for 10 to 15 minutes. Flip them over carefully with 2 forks and cook for another 10 minutes, until the sausage is cooked through and lightly crisped. If you desire a crispier shell, place the eggs under the broiler for about 3 to 5 minutes before serving.

NOTE: This recipe can also be used on the Carbohydrate Modification Plan as a breakfast entree.

Crispy Keto Beef Hash

MAKES 2 (½-CUP) SERVINGS

2 tablespoons extra-virgin olive oil

2 tablespoons diced onion

¼ teaspoon sea salt

⅛ teaspoon black pepper

¼ teaspoon dried oregano

⅛ teaspoon garlic powder

8 ounces ground beef

Beef hash—yes, it's what is for breakfast! I've doctored the original a little bit with the onion and some spices. It is a hearty meal any time of the day, too. Although there's fat in the ground beef already, I used some olive oil here as well. Researchers continue to uncover the hidden benefits of this oil, including that it may help prevent bone loss by aiding the osteoblasts (the cells) that help produce bone mass.

Heat the olive oil in a medium skillet over medium heat. Add the onion, salt, and pepper and sauté for 5 minutes, until tender. Add the oregano, garlic powder, and ground beef to the pan and stir well. Cook, stirring occasionally, for 10 minutes.

Press down on the hash, turn up the heat to high, and cook for 2 to 3 minutes, until the bottom is crisp and browned. Serve.

NOTE: This recipe can also be used on the Keto-Green Extreme Plan and the Carbohydrate Modification Plan as a breakfast entree.

ENTREES

Keto Texas Chili MAKES 3 TO 4 SERVINGS

2 tablespoons extra-virgin olive oil

½ medium onion, chopped

1 garlic clove, chopped

1 tablespoon chili powder

1 teaspoon chipotle powder or smoked paprika

1 teaspoon ground cumin

1 pound ground bison, beef, or turkey (preferably grass-fed)

1 ripe medium tomato, diced

1 tablespoon tomato paste

1 jalapeño pepper, sliced

½ cup low-sodium beef broth or bone broth

Sea salt and black pepper

This dish was so comforting in the winter of 2021, when I lived through Dallas's worst-ever snowstorm. I had to keep my horses warm, but I also had to keep my daughters warm and fed. This chili came to my rescue. It is the best winter meal. As a side note, traditional Texas chili has no beans, so it's perfect for the Carbohydrate Pause menu.

Heat the olive oil in a medium pot over medium heat. Add the onion and garlic and sauté about 3 minutes, until tender. Add the chili powder, chipotle powder, and cumin, stirring for a minute or so to extract the flavor from the spice. Add the meat. Use a spatula to crumble the meat and cook until no longer pink, 10 to 15 minutes.

Add the tomato and tomato paste, jalapeño, and broth. Bring to a boil and then reduce the heat to medium-low. Cover and simmer for at least 10 minutes, stirring occasionally. Season to taste with salt and pepper before serving.

NOTE: This recipe can also be used on the Carbohydrate Modification Plan as an entree.

Super Burgers

MAKES 6 SERVINGS

- 1 pound ground beef (preferably grass-fed)
- 8 ounces chicken livers, chopped
- 2 strips (no-sugar) bacon, cut into bits
- ½ teaspoon sea salt
- ¼ teaspoon black pepper
- 2 teaspoons ranch seasoning mix

I've started encouraging members of my Girlfriend Doctor Club to start eating more organ meats. Once a cherished food source, organ meats are overlooked today, but they are actually quite nutritious. Our hunter-gatherer ancestors knew this. They didn't just eat muscle meat; they consumed the organs too, such as liver, brains, and kidneys. In fact, the organs were highly prized. Let's bring them back, because organ meats are packed with nutrients such as vitamin B_{12} and folate, and they're also an excellent source of iron and protein. This recipe slips chicken livers in with the ground beef—and is a great dish to get you started on eating this amazing source of nutrition. This recipe makes more burgers than you likely will want at one time; just wrap and refrigerate the extras for other times.

Place the beef, chicken livers, bacon, salt, pepper, and seasoning mix in a food processor or blender, and pulse until well combined. Shape the mixture into 6 or more large patties.

Either heat a large skillet over medium-high heat or preheat a grill. Sauté or grill the burgers to the desired doneness, flipping once to brown on both sides. Serve alone—no buns!

NOTE: This recipe can also be used on the Carbohydrate Modification Plan as an entree.

Bacon-Wrapped Scallops

MAKES 2 SERVINGS

1 to 2 teaspoons extra-virgin olive oil

10 firm sea scallops (about 1 pound), patted dry

5 strips (no-sugar) bacon, cut in half lengthwise

Sea salt and black pepper

2 teaspoons drained capers

½ lemon, cut into wedges

I am a shellfish fan from way back. Here is one of my all-time favorites. It looks fancy enough to serve to guests at a dinner party—as either a main course or an appetizer—but it is easy enough to hold a more frequent slot in your recipe rotation.

Preheat the oven to 425°F. Brush a rimmed baking sheet with some of the olive oil.

Wrap each scallop with a slice of bacon and secure with a toothpick. Place the scallops on the prepared baking sheet and brush the tops with any remaining olive oil.

Season the scallops evenly with salt and pepper. Keep in mind that the bacon will provide some sodium, so go light on the salt. Bake for 15 minutes, until the scallops are opaque and the bacon is cooked.

Transfer the bacon-wrapped scallops to serving plates and spoon the capers over. Serve with a wedge of lemon.

NOTE: These scallops also are great with Sriracha and mayonnaise (or Vegenaise) dipping sauce on page 274.

NOTE: This recipe can also be used on the Keto-Green Extreme Plan (without the black pepper and the Sriracha dipping sauce) and the Carbohydrate Modification Plan as an entree.

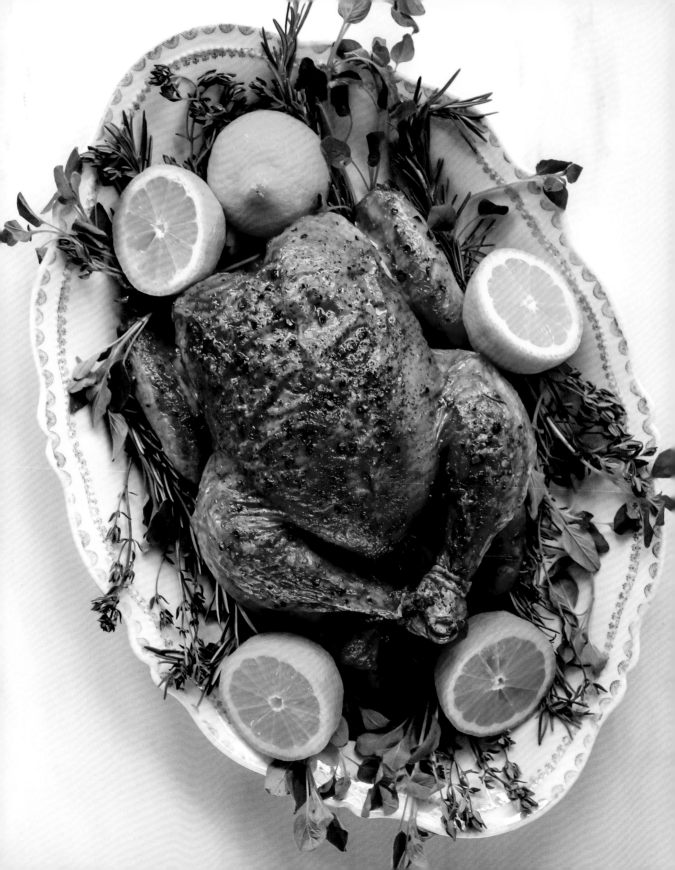

Classic Roast Chicken MAKES 3 TO 4 SERVINGS

1 (3½-pound) roasting chicken

1½ teaspoons sea salt, plus more for cavity

1 teaspoon black pepper, plus more for cavity

Juice of 1 large lemon

2 fresh oregano sprigs

2 fresh thyme sprigs

2 fresh rosemary sprigs

1 teaspoon garlic powder

½ teaspoon onion powder

½ teaspoon ground white pepper

3 tablespoons extra-virgin olive oil

For the perfect roast chicken dinner, try this family favorite. Its herby, lemon flavor will hook you. This recipe makes leftovers, too.

Preheat the oven to 400°F.

Season the cavity of the chicken with some salt and pepper. Place the chicken in a roasting pan. Pour the lemon juice into the pan, and stuff the squeezed lemon halves into the bird's cavity. Place the oregano, thyme, and rosemary sprigs in the cavity.

In a small bowl, combine the 1½ teaspoons salt, 1 teaspoon pepper, the garlic and onion powder, and white pepper. Evenly brush the olive oil all over the bird, then sprinkle on the spice mixture.

Place the chicken in the oven and roast for 1 hour, until the skin is crispy and the chicken is cooked through; an instant-read thermometer inserted in the thickest part of the breast should read 165°F.

Let the chicken rest for about 15 minutes before carving. Serve the chicken with bits of the crispy skin and drippings from the pan.

Pro tip: Reserve the bones and carcass for making chicken bone broth.

NOTE: This recipe can also be used on the Keto-Green Extreme Plan (without the black pepper or ground white pepper) and the Carbohydrate Modification Plan as an entree.

Beef Ribs with Bacon   MAKES 2 SERVINGS

1 teaspoon sea salt

1 teaspoon black pepper

1 teaspoon garlic powder

½ teaspoon chili powder

½ teaspoon ground cumin

½ teaspoon paprika

½ teaspoon dried oregano

1 pound beef back ribs

4 slices thick-cut (no-sugar) bacon

½ cup beef broth

1 tablespoon apple cider vinegar

Anyone for barbecue tonight? Here is a super-easy recipe you can make in your slow cooker early in the day, and it will be ready for dinner. If you don't have a slow cooker, or don't have all day, you can make it more quickly on the stovetop. The bacon sauté is the secret step that makes these ribs "a cut above." Bacon contains saturated fat; a little bit of it every now and then supports hormone production.

Oven Directions

Preheat the oven to 250°F.

In a small bowl, combine the salt, pepper, garlic powder, chili powder, cumin, paprika, and oregano. Use the spice mixture to evenly coat all sides of the ribs.

Over medium-high heat in an oven-safe Dutch oven, cook the bacon to desired doneness. (If you don't have an oven-safe Dutch oven, use a large skillet and transfer food to a casserole dish to roast.) Remove and drain on a plate lined with a paper towel.

Add the ribs to the Dutch oven and sear in the remaining bacon fat for about 5 minutes, until golden brown. Top with the broth and vinegar. Chop the bacon and add to the Dutch oven, then cover and place in the oven. Cook for 2 to 3 hours, until the meat is tender enough to fall off the bone.

Serve the ribs with spoonfuls of the cooking juices.

Slow Cooker Directions

Follow the oven directions for preparing the seasoning mix and coating the ribs, cooking the

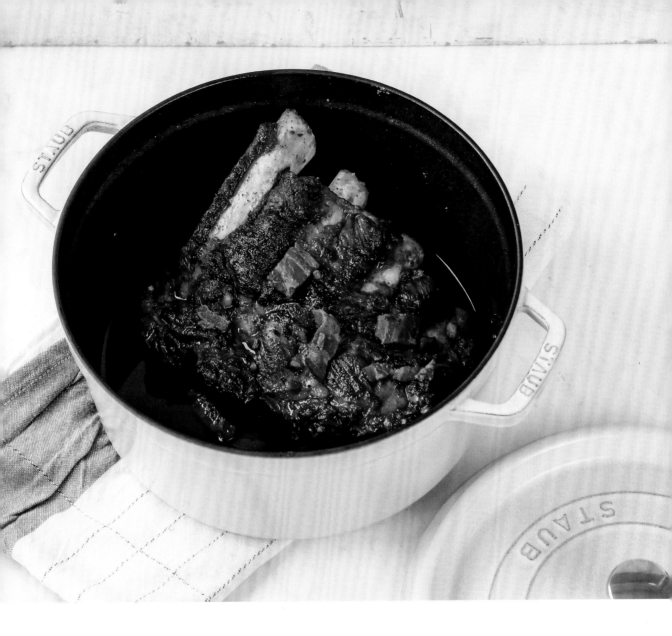

bacon, and browning the ribs. Transfer the ribs to a slow cooker and top with the broth and vinegar. Chop the bacon and add to the slow cooker as well, then cover and set to cook on high for 4 hours.

Serve the ribs with spoonfuls of the cooking juices.

NOTE: This recipe can also be used on the Carbohydrate Modification Plan as an entree.

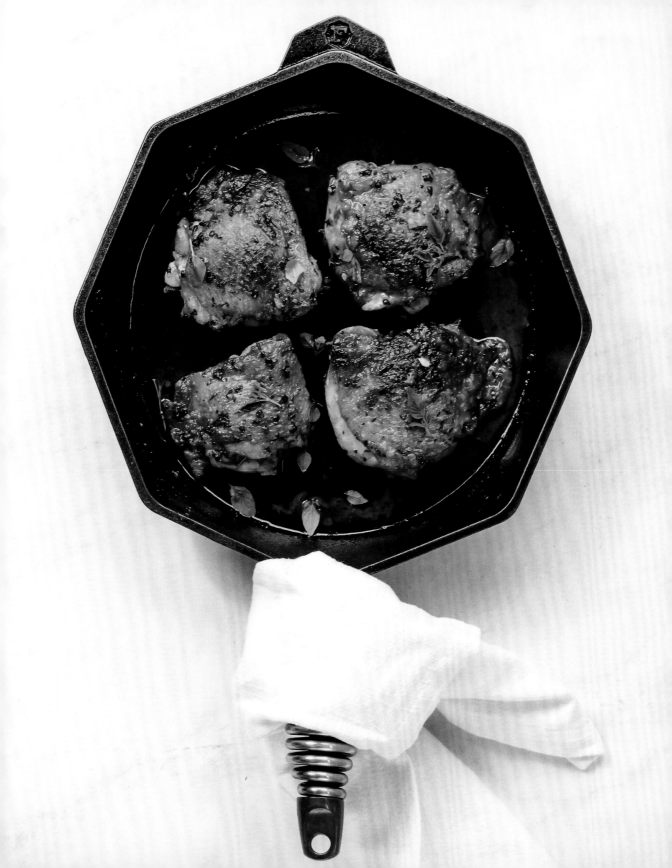

Crispy Chicken Thighs

MAKES 2 SERVINGS

1 tablespoon extra-virgin olive oil

1 pound skin-on, bone-in chicken thighs

1 teaspoon sea salt

1 teaspoon black pepper

2 tablespoons white wine vinegar or apple cider vinegar

2 tablespoons chicken broth or bone broth

1 teaspoon minced fresh oregano

My mom always cooked with a cast-iron skillet, and I do the same today. I love these skillets because they make anything cooked in them crispy and delicious. Also, they transfer easily from the stovetop to the oven. Of course, cooking with cast iron slightly increases the iron content of food, which is a plus for women who are deficient in this mineral.

Preheat the oven to 450°F.

Heat the olive oil in a large cast-iron skillet over medium-high heat (if you don't have a cast-iron skillet, use a large nonstick skillet and transfer the chicken mixture to a casserole dish before placing in the oven). Season the chicken thighs with salt and pepper, then place in the skillet skin side down. Cook for 8 to 10 minutes, until the skin is a deep golden brown and the fat has been rendered. The chicken should release easily from the pan when the skin is perfectly crisp; if it's still sticking, cook for another minute or two until it gives.

Remove the skillet from the heat and flip the chicken over so the skin is facing up. Pour in the vinegar, broth, and oregano. Place the skillet in the oven and cook for 15 to 20 minutes more, until the chicken is cooked through and an instant-read thermometer registers 165°F.

Serve the chicken thighs with the pan drippings spooned over.

NOTE: This recipe can also be used on the Keto-Green Extreme Plan (without the black pepper) and the Carbohydrate Modification Plan as an entree.

Kafta Kabobs

MAKES 2 SERVINGS

1 large onion, minced

4 tablespoons minced fresh parsley

1 pound ground lamb or beef (preferably grass-fed)

½ teaspoon sea salt

¼ teaspoon black pepper

¼ teaspoon ground allspice

6 wooden or metal skewers (if you're using wooden skewers, soak in water for 30 to 60 minutes ahead of using)

1 tablespoon chopped fresh mint (optional)

At home, we grill these all the time—a real family favorite. You can certainly make extra, and the kabobs can be frozen. That way, all you have to do is heat them up, and you've got a delicious meal in no time.

Preheat a grill on high or, if using an oven, preheat to 450°F.

In a medium bowl, combine the onion, parsley, lamb, salt and pepper, and allspice. Use your hands to blend the ingredients well.

Working in small portions, shape the meat mixture into 6 long sausage shapes about 6 inches in length. Thread the meat on the skewers but keep bare 1 inch from the skewer tip. Squeeze and mold each kabob on the skewer.

If using a grill, lightly oil it with a paper towel, holding it with tongs. Place the kabobs on the grill and cook, turning periodically, for 4 to 5 minutes per side. Be careful not to overcook.

If using the oven, lightly oil a baking sheet and arrange the kabobs on the sheet. Roast on the middle rack of the oven for 12 to 15 minutes, turning the kabobs over halfway through the roasting time.

NOTE: This recipe can also be used on the Keto-Green Extreme Plan without the black pepper and allspice, and on the Carbohydrate Modification Plan as an entree.

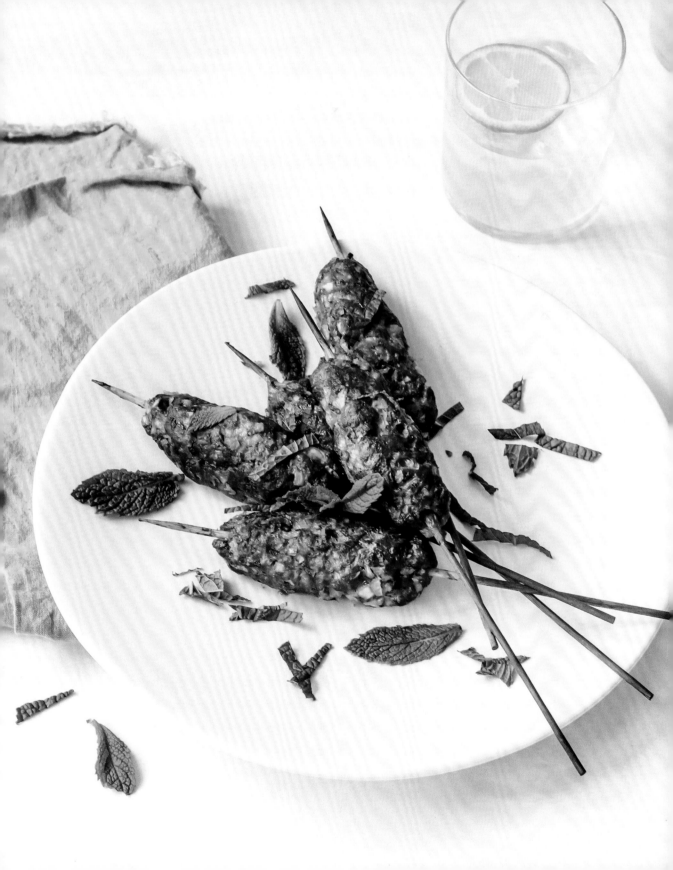

Vinegar-Poached Herby Fish

MAKES 2 SERVINGS

1 tablespoon extra-virgin olive oil

1 garlic clove, minced

½ medium shallot, minced

1 teaspoon minced fresh thyme

1 teaspoon minced fresh oregano

3 tablespoons white wine vinegar

¼ cup chicken broth or bone broth

2 cod fillets, 4 to 6 ounces each (or other firm-fleshed white fish)

Sea salt and black pepper

1 tablespoon chopped fresh parsley

Fish cooks so easily and so quickly, especially when poached. My go-to poaching liquid is a broth because the flavored liquid imparts even more flavor to the fish. It also contains healing, alkalinizing minerals.

Heat the olive oil in a large skillet over medium-high heat. Add the garlic and shallot and cook for 3 to 4 minutes, until the shallot is translucent. Add the thyme and oregano, and cook for another minute, then add the vinegar and broth. Bring to a boil, then reduce the heat to medium.

Season the fish with salt and pepper on both sides, then gently add to the skillet. Cover and cook for 4 to 5 minutes, until the fish is opaque and flakes easily with a fork.

Serve the fish with spoonfuls of the pan juices and sprinkle the parsley on top.

NOTE: This recipe can also be used on the Keto-Green Extreme Plan (without the black pepper) and the Carbohydrate Modification Plan as an entree.

Garlic and Herbed Leg of Lamb

MAKES 3-4 SERVINGS

2 tablespoons extra-virgin olive oil

½ leg of lamb (3 to 4 pounds), patted dry

2 teaspoons sea salt

1½ teaspoons black pepper

1½ teaspoons garlic powder

1 cup beef broth or bone broth

2 tablespoons apple cider vinegar

2 fresh oregano sprigs

2 fresh thyme sprigs

1 fresh rosemary sprig

1 bay leaf

For a change of pace, try lamb occasionally. This herby preparation will get you started. Among animal proteins, lamb is richer in iron than chicken or fish. After menopause, your daily recommended intake for iron goes from 18 milligrams to just 8 milligrams. That means it's a lot easier to meet your iron needs through diet alone, and lamb can help do that. But no matter what your current life stage, it's a good idea to include iron-friendly foods in your diet, because iron supports blood health and energy metabolism. This recipe can be made in the oven or in a slow cooker.

Oven Directions

Preheat the oven to 350°F.

Evenly brush the olive oil on the lamb and sprinkle with the salt, pepper, and garlic powder.

Place the lamb in a roasting pan, fat side up, and add the broth, vinegar, and herb sprigs.

Roast the lamb for 60 to 90 minutes, until an instant-read thermometer inserted in the thickest part registers 135° F. Let the meat rest for at least 15 minutes. Then slice and serve with the pan juices.

Slow Cooker Directions

Season the lamb evenly with the salt, pepper, and garlic powder.

(recipe continues)

Heat the olive oil in a large skillet over medium-high heat. Add the lamb and sear for about 5 minutes on all sides, until golden brown. Transfer the lamb to a slow cooker and add the broth, vinegar, and herb sprigs. Cover and set to cook on high for 4 hours. Let the meat rest for at least 15 minutes. Then slice and serve with the juices from the cooker.

NOTE: This recipe can also be used on the Keto-Green Extreme Plan (without the black pepper) and the Carbohydrate Modification Plan as an entree.

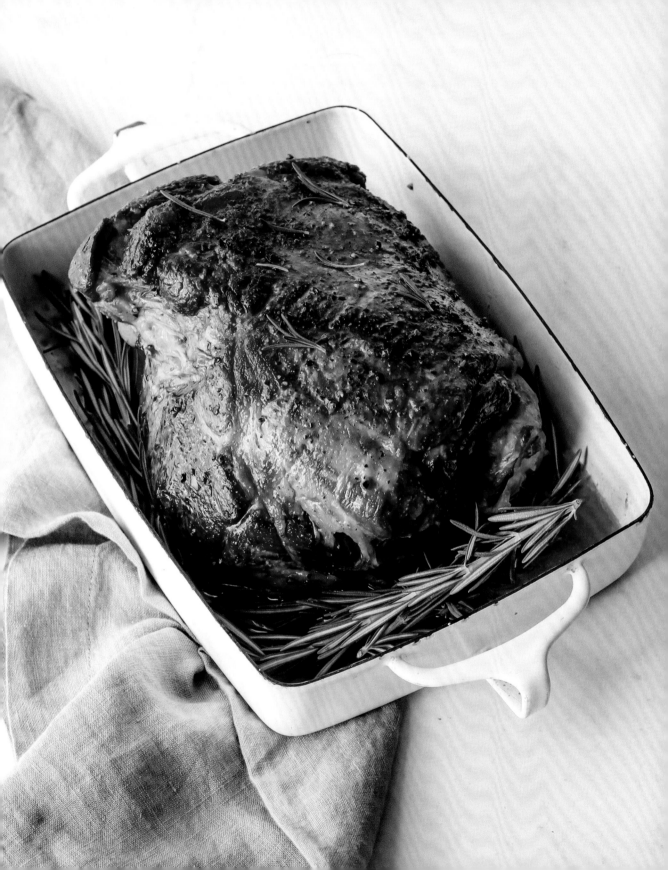

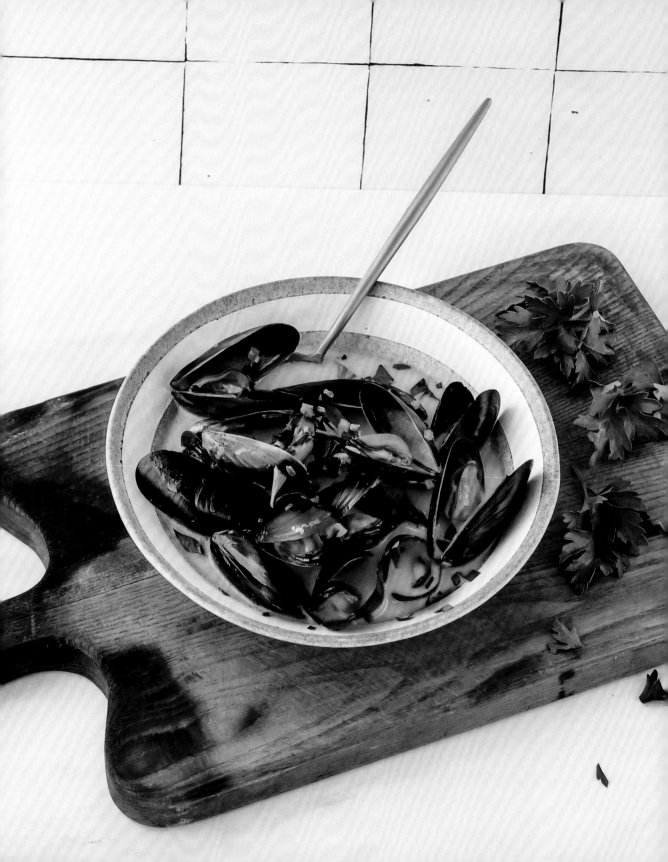

Creamy Coconut-Saffron Mussels

MAKES 2 SERVINGS

Pinch of saffron threads

1 pound mussels in the shell, washed

3 tablespoons coconut oil

1 small shallot, minced

2 garlic cloves, minced

2 tablespoons fresh lemon juice

¼ cup chicken broth or bone broth

½ (14-ounce) can full-fat coconut milk

1 teaspoon sea salt

1 teaspoon black pepper

2 tablespoons chopped fresh parsley

Here's a chance for you to step out of your kitchen comfort zone and try cooking mussels, if you've never done so before. This recipe is one of the quickest shellfish preparations anywhere. The lemony sauce is the "icing on the cake," so to speak. And here's a health fact on saffron: it offers an antidepressant benefit. Studies have found that saffron prevents the depletion of serotonin, that feel-good neurotransmitter that helps stabilize mood.

Using a mortar and pestle or other heavy utensil, grind saffron threads into a powder. Pour ¼ cup hot water over them and set aside.

Rinse mussels under cold water and remove any beards.

Heat coconut oil in a large pot over medium-high heat. Once oil is melted and hot, add shallot and garlic to the pot. Stir for 3 to 4 minutes or until shallot is translucent and garlic is golden.

Add lemon juice, broth, coconut milk, and saffron water to the pot. Stir and scrape up any bits stuck to the bottom of the pot. Then add mussels and toss to coat in sauce. Season with salt and pepper to taste. Cover and steam for 5 to 6 minutes or until all the mussels have opened.

Serve mussels with the sauce and fresh parsley on top.

NOTE: This recipe can also be used on the Carbohydrate Modification Plan as an entree.

Southwestern Spiced Pork Tenderloin

MAKES 2 SERVINGS

1½ teaspoons sea salt

½ teaspoon black pepper

1 teaspoon garlic powder

1 teaspoon paprika

½ teaspoon chili powder

½ teaspoon dried oregano

½ teaspoon onion powder

¼ teaspoon cayenne

2 tablespoons extra-virgin olive oil

1 (2-pound) pork tenderloin

¼ cup chicken broth or bone broth

2 tablespoons apple cider vinegar

1 bay leaf

Pork tenderloin, like most other pork cuts, can be incredibly delicious, juicy, and tender. But because it is a lean cut, you have to cook it correctly, or else it can go from perfectly cooked to overcooked pretty quickly. Preparing the recipe in a slow cooker solves this problem because the tenderloin is braised slowly in liquid. Of course, you can also cook it in the oven, with good results.

Oven Directions

Preheat the oven to 350°F.

In a small bowl, combine the salt, pepper, garlic powder, paprika, chili powder, oregano, onion powder, and cayenne. Rub the pork generously on all sides with the spice mixture.

Heat the olive oil in a large skillet over high heat. Add the pork and sear for 5 minutes on all sides, until browned.

Transfer the pork to a rimmed baking sheet. Pour the broth and vinegar into the pan, add the bay leaf, and tent with aluminum foil. Roast for 25 to 30 minutes, until an instant-read thermometer inserted into the thickest part reads 150°F.

Let the pork rest for about 15 minutes before slicing. Remove the bay leaf. Serve the pork slices with some of the cooking juices spooned over.

Slow Cooker Directions

Follow the directions for oven roasting by rubbing the pork with the spice mixture, then searing the pork in the skillet on the stovetop.

Transfer the pork to a slow cooker, pour in the broth and vinegar, and add the bay leaf. Cover the cooker and set to cook on high for 4 hours. Let the pork rest for about 15 minutes before slicing. Remove the bay leaf. Serve the pork slices with some of the cooking juices spooned over.

NOTE: This recipe can also be used on the Carbohydrate Modification Plan as an entree.

Balsamic-Oregano Beef Heart

1 beef heart (about 3 pounds), patted dry, cut open and arteries removed, and excess fat discarded (or ask your butcher to do this)

2 teaspoons sea salt, or more as needed

2 teaspoons minced fresh oregano

4 tablespoons extra-virgin olive oil

½ cup balsamic vinegar (sugar-free)

1 teaspoon black pepper, or more as needed

1 teaspoon garlic powder

2 tablespoons extra-virgin olive oil

¼ cup beef broth or bone broth

NOTE: This recipe can also be used on the Keto-Green Extreme Plan (without the black pepper) and the Carbohydrate Modification Plan as an entree.

There's no reason to shy away from organ meats. They've been traditional medicine for centuries. If you've never tried any of the organ meats, this recipe is a great intro. It uses mineral-packed beef heart, which tastes like steak.

Season the beef heart with 1 teaspoon of the salt and 1 teaspoon of the oregano. Let sit at least 20 minutes for the seasonings to be absorbed.

Pour 2 tablespoons of the olive oil and the balsamic vinegar into a zippered plastic bag. Add the heart and massage the bag to coat the meat with the marinade. Place in the refrigerator to marinate for at least 4 hours or overnight. Turn the bag every hour or so to ensure even marinating.

Allow the meat to warm to room temperature before cooking. Then, take the meat out of the bag and pat dry. Reserve the marinade. Season the meat evenly with the remaining teaspoon salt and the remaining teaspoon oregano, along with the pepper and garlic powder.

Heat the remaining 2 tablespoons olive oil in a large cast-iron skillet over medium-high heat. Add the heart and cook for 5 minutes per side, until evenly golden brown. Let the meat rest on a platter for 20 minutes before slicing.

Meanwhile, make the sauce. Pour half the reserved marinade into the skillet along with the broth. Bring to a boil, then reduce the heat to medium-low and cook for 15 minutes to reduce the sauce by half. Taste and adjust the salt and pepper as needed.

Thinly slice the beef heart and serve with the sauce.

Crispy Skin Salmon

MAKES 2 SERVINGS

2 salmon fillets, 4 to 6 ounces each, patted dry, skin left on

2 tablespoons extra-virgin olive oil

½ teaspoon sea salt

½ teaspoon black pepper

½ teaspoon garlic powder

½ teaspoon onion powder

½ teaspoon paprika

¼ teaspoon dried oregano

The skin of a salmon fillet contains the highest concentration of omega-3 fatty acids on the whole fish. There's strong proof that these fatty acids can protect you from heart disease, restore hormone balance, and even help your skin look more youthful. The reason for all these benefits—and more—is that omega-3 fats calm any inflammation, the culprit behind many diseases and a contributor to aging. So, say yes to salmon skin.

Lightly brush both sides of the fillets with some of the olive oil and evenly season with the salt, pepper, garlic and onion powder, paprika, and oregano.

Heat the remaining olive oil in a large skillet over medium-high heat. Add the salmon fillets, skin side down, and cook for 2 minutes. Reduce the heat to medium and cook for another 5 minutes. While the salmon cooks, occasionally press down with a spatula so the skin comes into full contact with the hot pan. Flip the fillets over and then turn off the heat.

Allow the salmon to finish cooking in the hot pan for 30 to 60 seconds. Then transfer the fillets to serving plates.

NOTE: This recipe can also be used on the Keto-Green Extreme Plan (without the black pepper and paprika) and the Carbohydrate Modification Plan as an entree.

Ghee-Basted Pork Chops MAKES 2 SERVINGS

2 garlic cloves, grated on a box grater

2 teaspoons minced fresh thyme

2 teaspoons minced fresh rosemary

¼ cup apple cider vinegar

2 tablespoons extra-virgin olive oil

2 thick-cut, bone-in pork chops (6 ounces each)

Sea salt and black pepper

2 tablespoons ghee (clarified butter)

Pork chops are the most popular cut of pork and are the least intimidating because they are so easy to prepare. This version is one of the easiest and you'll love the way the herbs bring out the flavor of the pork. Along with apple cider vinegar, they help make this meat dish more alkalinizing.

In a small bowl, whisk together the garlic, thyme, rosemary, vinegar, and olive oil. Pour into a zippered plastic bag. Season the chops with salt and pepper, then add to the bag with the marinade. Massage the bag a bit to coat the chops well. Place the bag in the refrigerator to marinate for at least 2 hours or overnight.

Thirty minutes before you plan to cook the pork chops, remove them from the refrigerator to warm to room temperature.

Heat the ghee in a large skillet over medium-high heat. Pat the chops dry, then add to the skillet and sear for 5 to 6 minutes per side; do not touch pork chops while they sear. Using tongs, flip the chops and use a spoon to baste them with the pan juices. Cook for another 5 minutes, continuing to baste.

Let the chops rest for 5 to 10 minutes, then slice and serve.

NOTE: This recipe can also be used on the Carbohydrate Modification Plan as an entree.

Bacon-Wrapped Chicken Tenders MAKES 2 SERVINGS

½ teaspoon sea salt

½ teaspoon black pepper

½ teaspoon garlic powder

½ teaspoon paprika

½ teaspoon dried thyme

8 chicken tenders (about 1 pound)

8 slices (no-sugar) bacon

I love wrapping foods in bacon! The bacon just takes the flavor of those foods up a notch, especially when paired with herbs and spices. I'm always looking for new ways to prepare chicken, and this recipe is one of the best I've found.

Preheat the oven to 425°F. Line a baking sheet with parchment paper.

In a small bowl, combine the salt, pepper, garlic powder, paprika, and thyme. Evenly season the chicken with the spice blend. Wrap each piece of chicken with 1 strip of bacon.

Arrange the chicken pieces on the baking sheet and bake for 35 to 40 minutes, until the bacon is crisp and the chicken is cooked through. Serve.

NOTE: This recipe can also be used on the Keto-Green Extreme Plan (without the black pepper and paprika) and the Carbohydrate Modification Plan as an entree.

Ginger-Soy Shredded Beef

MAKES 2 SERVINGS

½ cup beef broth or bone broth

2 tablespoons coconut aminos

1 tablespoon grated fresh ginger

1 tablespoon toasted sesame oil

1 teaspoon white sesame seeds

2 tablespoons extra-virgin olive oil

1 boneless beef chuck roast, about 1½ pounds

Sea salt and black pepper

1 teaspoon garlic powder

NOTE: This recipe can also be used on the Carbohydrate Modification Plan as an entree.

Here's an amazing beef recipe with Asian flair, thanks to a touch of ginger. Fresh ginger is a super herb with a long list of health benefits. Its main active compound is gingerol, which is responsible for most of the root's medicinal properties, including the fact that ginger is an anti-inflammatory and antioxidant herb. One of ginger's outstanding and most well-known benefits is that it soothes the stomach. This dish can be made either in the oven or in a slow cooker.

Oven Directions

Preheat the oven to 350°F.

In a medium bowl, whisk together the broth, coconut aminos, ginger, sesame oil, and sesame seeds.

Heat the olive oil in a large oven-safe Dutch oven over medium-high heat. (If you don't have an oven-safe Dutch oven, transfer food to casserole dish before placing in the oven.) Season both sides of the beef with salt and pepper and the garlic powder, then sear both sides of the meat for about 5 minutes, until golden. Pour the broth mixture over the top, cover the Dutch oven, and place in the oven to cook for 15 minutes. Then reduce the oven to 250°F and cook for another 1½ to 2 hours, until the meat is tender and breaks apart easily.

Allow to cool slightly, then place the meat in a large bowl. Shred it with 2 forks, then serve with the pan juices.

Slow Cooker Directions

Follow the directions for oven preparation and heat the olive oil and brown the meat in a large skillet.

Combine the broth, coconut aminos, ginger, sesame oil, and sesame seeds in a slow cooker. Stir, then add the beef roast. Cover and set to cook on high for 3 to 4 hours, until the meat is tender and falls apart. Allow to cool slightly, then transfer to a large bowl and shred the meat with 2 forks. Serve with juices from the cooker.

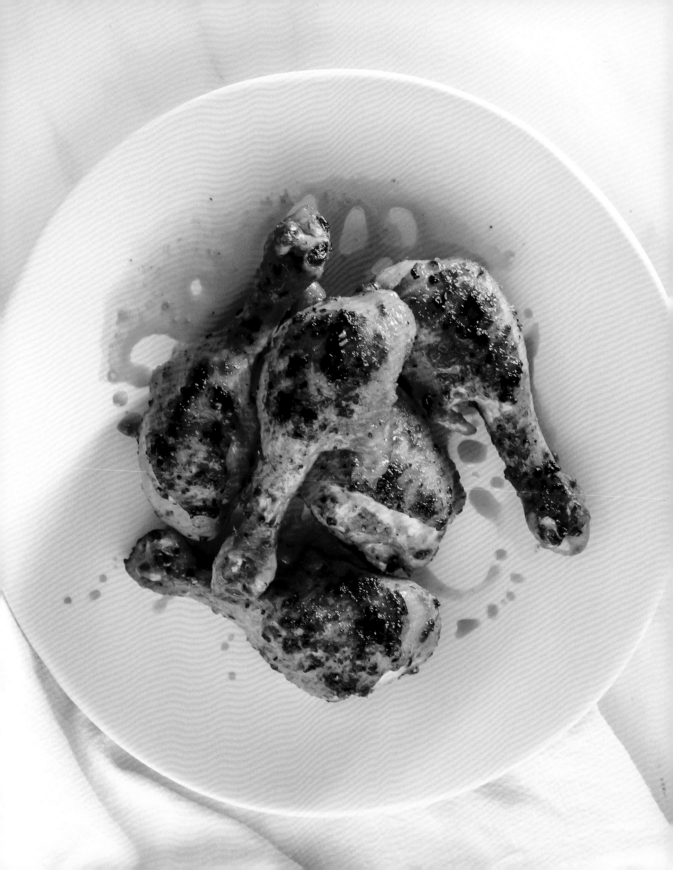

Easy Roasted Drumsticks

MAKES 2 SERVINGS

1 teaspoon sea salt, or more as needed

1 teaspoon black pepper

1 teaspoon garlic powder

½ teaspoon onion powder

½ teaspoon paprika

¼ teaspoon dried thyme

1 teaspoon grated lemon zest

2 teaspoons fresh lemon juice

2 tablespoons extra-virgin olive oil

1 pound chicken drumsticks

I do love the dark meat of chicken drumsticks—so moist and juicy. Compared with a chicken's white meat, the dark meat is higher in iron, zinc, selenium, and B vitamins, all of which are important for building your immune defenses and energy systems.

Preheat the oven to 425°F. Line a baking sheet with parchment paper.

In a small bowl, whisk together the salt, pepper, garlic and onion powder, paprika, thyme, lemon zest and juice, and olive oil.

Place the chicken in a medium bowl and drizzle the mixture over. Toss the drumsticks in the seasoning until evenly coated. Arrange the drumsticks on the baking sheet and roast for 35 to 40 minutes, until the skin is crispy and golden and meat is cooked through. An instant-read thermometer inserted in the thickest part should be 165°F.

Transfer the drumsticks to serving plates. Season with additional salt, if desired.

NOTE: This recipe can also be used on the Keto-Green Extreme Plan (without the black pepper and paprika) and the Carbohydrate Modification Plan as an entree.

Ribeye Steak with Spiced Ghee

MAKES 2 SERVINGS

For the spiced ghee

- 4 tablespoons ghee (clarified butter), at room temperature
- ¼ teaspoon sea salt
- ¼ teaspoon black pepper
- 1 teaspoon chopped fresh parsley
- ½ teaspoon chopped fresh thyme
- ½ teaspoon chopped fresh oregano

For the steaks

- 2 bone-in ribeye steaks (about 6 ounces each)
- 1 teaspoon sea salt
- 1 teaspoon black pepper
- 1 teaspoon garlic powder
- 1 teaspoon chopped fresh rosemary
- ½ teaspoon chopped fresh oregano
- 1 tablespoon extra-virgin olive oil

NOTE: This recipe can also be used on the Carbohydrate Modification Plan as an entree.

This steak takes a little extra prep, but it's worth it. A standout herb here is the parsley. Not only can it help fight menopause symptoms but it may also reduce the risk of osteoporosis.

Make the spiced ghee. In a food processor, combine the ingredients for the spiced ghee, pureeing until smooth. Scoop the mixture onto a piece of parchment paper and roll into a log. Place in the refrigerator to chill, at least 30 minutes or up to a week in advance.

Season the steaks. Rub the steaks evenly on all sides with the salt, pepper, garlic powder, and fresh herbs. Place on a small baking sheet or plate, cover with plastic wrap, and place in the refrigerator to season and tenderize for at least 2 hours or up to 2 days before cooking.

Cook and serve the steaks. An hour before you plan to cook, remove the steaks from the refrigerator so they can warm to room temperature.

Heat the olive oil and 1 tablespoon of the spiced ghee in a large skillet over medium-high heat. Add the steaks and cook for 5 minutes, until golden and caramelized on the bottom. Flip the steaks and cook on the other side for another 4 to 5 minutes, until golden and caramelized. Using a spoon, continually baste the steaks with the pan juices as they cook to preferred doneness.

Let the steaks rest for 5 to 10 minutes, then slice and serve with a pat of the spiced ghee on top.

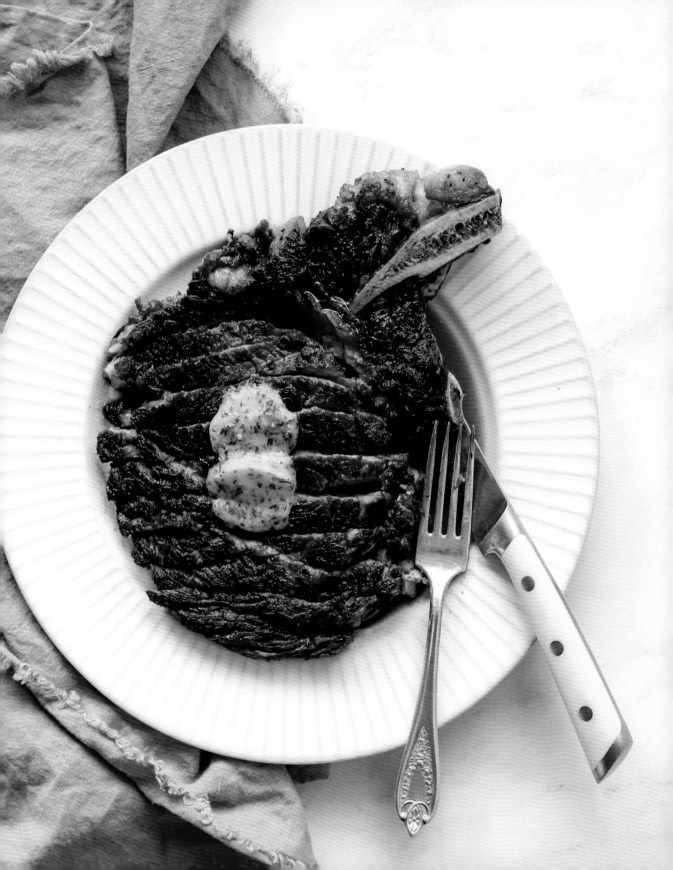

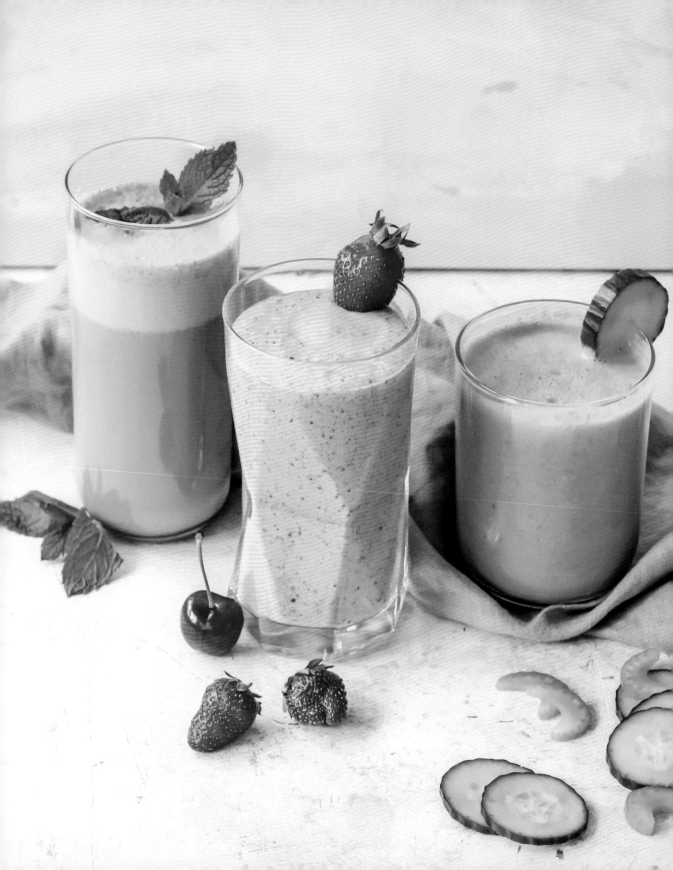

CHAPTER 12

The Keto-Green Cleanse Recipes

To view videos of the preparation of some of the recipes in this plan, go to dranna.com/menupause-extras.

Lemon Liver Flush

MAKES 6 SERVINGS

I recommend having this blend first thing in the morning for detoxification. The combination of olive oil and lemon is known to help cleanse the liver and gallbladder, clearing away any stored bile, cholesterol, and gallstones.

1 lemon, quartered

1 quart (4 cups) filtered water, at room temperature or chilled

2 tablespoons extra-virgin olive oil

2 drops stevia (optional)

¼ teaspoon vanilla extract (optional)

Place the lemon in a blender (Vitamix or comparable). Add the water, olive oil, and the stevia and vanilla (if using) and blend for 60 seconds. Strain through a fine-mesh strainer into a glass and enjoy. The drink will be creamy and tart.

Option: If you are time-crunched like I am, make enough in your blender for the week and store them in three small Mason jars in your refrigerator. All you have to do is take one out and chug it down. Alternatively, just do a shot of olive oil with the juice of a squeeze of lemon.

Collagen Hot Chocolate

MAKES 1 SERVING

As I mentioned earlier, collagen powder is an anti-aging protein in so many ways. In addition to putting it into your smoothies, here's another delicious way to serve up its healing power—in a warm mug of chocolaty goodness.

1½ cups unsweetened non-dairy milk (almond, cashew, or coconut)

Monk fruit, stevia, or cinnamon to taste

1 tablespoon cacao powder

¼ teaspoon vanilla extract

1 to 2 scoops (about 20 grams) collagen powder

In a small saucepan, heat the milk over medium heat but do not allow it to boil. Add the monk fruit, stevia, or cinnamon, cacao, and vanilla, and whisk thoroughly. Add the collagen and whisk until dissolved. Transfer to a mug and enjoy!

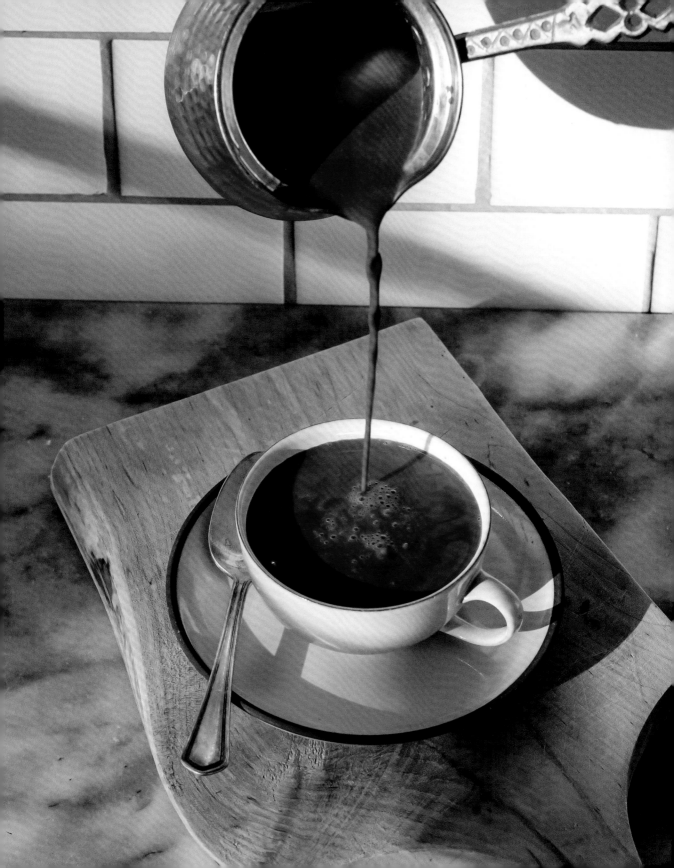

Mighty Maca Margarita

MAKES 1 SERVING

I'm always looking for new ways to use maca in recipes, and this one is both delicious and refreshing. Supplementing with maca is vital to maintaining hormone health and alkalinity. Highly nutritious, maca boosts libido, relieves menopause symptoms, improves mood and memory, and eases fatigue, among other benefits.

3 tablespoons fresh lemon juice

2 scoops Mighty Maca Plus, or 1 teaspoon maca root powder

1 cup organic sugar-free margarita mix

Crushed ice

Pour the lemon juice, maca, and margarita mix into a shaker. Shake well. Place some crushed ice in a 10-ounce margarita glass. Pour mix over ice. Enjoy this in mid-afternoon as a refreshing pick-me-up.

Option: Add sparkling water instead of margarita mix.

Creamy Vanilla-Mint Shake

MAKES 1 SERVING

Fresh mint brings this shake to life. Mint is rich in many nutrients, especially disease-fighting antioxidants, and is known to boost brain health. One of its other benefits is in digestive health. It soothes both irritable bowel syndrome and indigestion. Mint is so easy to add to your diet.

1½ cups unsweetened almond milk

1 cup baby spinach

10 to 12 fresh mint leaves

1 tablespoon almond butter

¼ teaspoon vanilla extract

Place the almond milk, spinach, mint, almond butter, and vanilla in a blender and blend well. Pour into a glass and enjoy.

Drinkable Berry Yogurt

MAKES 1 SERVING

Eaten for thousands of years, yogurt is one of the most popular fermented products in the world, made by adding live bacteria to a dairy or non-dairy base. The power of yogurt lies in its beneficial bacteria. It functions as a probiotic, providing healing benefits for the gut. It is incredibly easy to make your own yogurt, and this recipe shows you how.

1 (14-ounce) can full-fat coconut milk

2 capsules probiotics

1 cup berries of choice, fresh or frozen

Pour the coconut milk into a large glass container. Sprinkle in the probiotics and stir well to combine. Place in oven, turn on the oven light, and leave overnight. In the morning, place the yogurt in a blender and add the berries; blend until smooth. (Alternatively, use an immersion blender right in the glass container.) Refrigerate to chill, if desired, or enjoy immediately!

Green Goodness Smoothie

MAKES 1 SERVING

Here is a true alkalinizing smoothie. Also, you get your protein from the seeds and nut milk. The MCT oil helps your body get into the fat-burning state of ketosis—plus it keeps hunger pangs at bay.

½ cup unsweetened almond or coconut milk

1 celery stalk, chopped

½ medium cucumber, chopped

1 handful fresh spinach or other greens

¼ cup fresh parsley

2 tablespoons hemp seeds or flax seeds

1 tablespoon MCT or coconut oil

½ tablespoon fresh lemon juice

Dash of ground cinnamon and nutmeg

Liquid stevia (optional)

¼ avocado, cubed (optional)

6 ice cubes

Place the smoothie ingredients in a blender, and blend well. Pour into a glass and enjoy.

Lemon-Ginger Zinger MAKES 1 SERVING

If you can find them, go with dandelion greens as your first choice in this refreshing drink. They are among the best detoxifying veggies you can consume. Other attributes of the dandelion plant are its ability to lower cholesterol, blood pressure, and inflammation. All these benefits are probably due to the fact that dandelion is a superior source of vitamins A, C, E, and K, along with many minerals. The lemon and ginger in this recipe help cut the sometimes bitter taste of these healthful greens.

½ cup dandelion greens or kale

½ cup fresh spinach

1 (2-inch) slice fresh ginger

½ lemon, quartered (for easier blending)

½ avocado, cubed

1½ cups water

1 to 2 scoops Mighty Maca Plus, or 1 teaspoon maca root powder

Place zinger ingredients in a blender, and blend well. Pour into a glass and enjoy.

Nutty-for-Green Smoothie

MAKES 1 SERVING

At the heart of this smoothie is the cashew nut. Cashews have such a creamy, sweet taste—which is why I love using them in recipes. Beyond their yumminess, cashews are low in sugar and high in protein. They've been linked to benefits like weight loss, improved blood sugar control, and a healthier heart.

1 cup unsweetened cashew milk

1 cup fresh spinach

¼ avocado, cubed

8 to 10 unsalted cashews

1 tablespoon unsweetened coconut flakes

1 teaspoon ground cinnamon

1 to 2 scoops Mighty Maca Plus, or 1 teaspoon maca root powder

Place the smoothie ingredients in a blender, and blend well. Pour into a glass and enjoy.

NOTE: This recipe can also be used on the Carbohydrate Modification Plan as a breakfast entree.

Blender Green Veggie Juice

MAKES 1 SERVING

To enjoy green juice and reap its health and alkalinizing benefits, you don't need a juicer. A blender works fine—actually better. Blending these ingredients preserves all the fiber, which is lost when you juice. This juice may help with bloating, too, because cucumber and celery are natural diuretics.

1½ cups water

½ medium cucumber, chopped

2 celery stalks, chopped

½ green apple, chopped

½ lemon

1 handful of fresh spinach

1 scoop Dr. Anna's Keto-Green Meal Replacement mix or substitute (see page 120)

1 to 2 scoops Mighty Maca Plus, or 1 teaspoon maca root powder

Place the water, cucumber, celery, apple, lemon, spinach, Meal Replacement mix, and Mighty Maca Plus in a blender, and blend well. Pour into a glass and enjoy.

Pineapple-Pepper Green Juice

MAKES 1 SERVING

Just about everything in this blender juice is good for your gut—ginger with its phytonutrients, kale with its prebiotics to feed your friendly gut bacteria, and pineapple to help with digestion. Beyond the nutrition, this beverage is just plain delicious!

1 cup coconut water

2 teaspoons fresh lemon juice

1 (1-inch) piece fresh ginger

1 cup stemmed kale leaves

½ cup frozen pineapple chunks

1 tablespoon MCT or coconut oil

Pinch of cayenne

Place the ingredients in a blender, and blend well. Pour into a glass and enjoy.

Piña Wholada,
opposite

Pumpkin Protein
Shake, page 240

Peach Melba Smoothie,
opposite

Peach Melba Smoothie

MAKES 1 SERVING

Peach Melba is a dessert of peaches and raspberry sauce that was invented in 1892 by a French chef to honor an Australian soprano named Nellie Melba. It has been popular ever since. I've turned it into a smoothie that I hope will be popular with you, too! Raspberries, aside from their strong antioxidant and vitamin C content, are known for their anti-inflammatory properties. As for peaches, they are just plain delicious— something I know well because I lived in Georgia, the Peach State, for so long.

1½ cups unsweetened almond milk or coconut milk

½ cup chopped frozen peaches

½ cup frozen raspberries

1 cup stemmed kale leaves

¼ medium cucumber, cubed

2 tablespoons hemp seeds or freshly ground flax seeds

1 to 2 scoops Mighty Maca Plus, or 1 teaspoon maca root powder

Place the smoothie ingredients in a blender, and blend well. Pour into a glass and enjoy.

Piña Wholada

MAKES 1 SERVING

Ah, a piña colada—a delightful blend of coconut and pineapple. I recommend pineapple frequently because it contains a group of digestive enzymes called bromelain that help break down protein into its building blocks, including amino acids. This aids the digestion and absorption of protein.

1 cup unsweetened coconut milk

2 tablespoons full-fat coconut cream (skimmed from the top of the chilled can of coconut cream)

¼ cup frozen pineapple chunks

Handful of fresh spinach or other greens

1 scoop Dr. Anna's Keto-Green Meal Replacement mix or substitute (see page 120)

1 tablespoon MCT or coconut oil

1 teaspoon banana extract or vanilla extract

1 to 2 scoops Mighty Maca Plus, or 1 teaspoon maca root powder

Place the ingredients in a blender, and blend well. Pour into a glass and enjoy.

Pumpkin Protein Shake

MAKES 1 SERVING

I have a love affair with pumpkin puree and am always on the lookout for ways to use it. It is popular around the holidays, but I enjoy it year-round. As this recipe shows, you can freeze it for your smoothies, making them almost like pumpkin ice cream. Pumpkin flesh is packed with powerful nutrients that help reduce the risk of high blood pressure, abnormal cholesterol, and Type 2 diabetes.

1 cup unsweetened almond or coconut milk

¼ cup canned pumpkin puree, frozen if desired

1½ teaspoons pumpkin pie spice

1 scoop Dr. Anna's Keto-Green Meal Replacement mix or substitute (see page 120)

1 tablespoon MCT or coconut oil

1 teaspoon vanilla extract

1 to 2 scoops Mighty Maca Plus, or 1 teaspoon maca root powder

Place the ingredients in a blender, and blend well. Pour into a glass and enjoy.

Pork Bone Broth

MAKES ABOUT 1½ QUARTS

The first time I made broth from pork bones, I was surprised by how much collagen the bones yielded. Once the broth cooled, I put it in my fridge, and it was thick jelly the next day. The more a broth gels, the more collagen it contains.

2 pounds pork bones (from ribs or ham hocks)

6 garlic cloves, halved

1 (2-inch) slice fresh ginger

4 scallions (green parts only), halved

2 celery stalks, roughly chopped

2 tablespoons apple cider vinegar

Large pinch of sea salt

6 cups water

Place the bones, garlic, ginger, scallion greens, celery, vinegar, and salt in a large pot. Add the water and cover the pot. Bring to a boil over high heat, then reduce the heat to low and cook for 12 hours.

Strain the broth through a coarse-mesh strainer or colander and season with salt to taste. Let the broth cool in the fridge, then skim the fat off the top.

Roasted Chicken Bone Broth

MAKES 2 QUARTS

Carcass from 1 roasted chicken, including skin if possible

1 medium onion, quartered

2 medium carrots, cut into 2-inch pieces (unpeeled)

2 celery stalks, cut into 2-inch pieces, including leaves

2 garlic cloves, smashed

1 bay leaf

Handful of fresh parsley

2 teaspoons dried sage

2 teaspoons black pepper

2 tablespoons apple cider vinegar

1 teaspoon ground turmeric

2½ quarts water

Sea salt

Never toss out a chicken bone! Collect those bones by storing in the freezer. When you get a bunch, start making your broth. Have you ever wondered why bone broth recipes specify vinegar? Because it helps the bones release their minerals into the broth.

Add the carcass, onion, carrots, celery, garlic, bay leaf, parsley, sage, pepper, vinegar, and turmeric to a large stockpot. Add the water, cover the pot, and bring to a boil over high heat, then reduce the heat to low and simmer for 12 hours. To make broth in a slow cooker, see page 228 of *The Hormone Fix*.

Remove the bones and vegetables from the broth and discard. Strain the broth through a coarse-mesh sieve or colander and then season with salt to taste. Let the broth cool; refrigerate and then skim the fat off the top.

Dr. Anna's Beef Bone Broth MAKES ABOUT 2 QUARTS

2 carrots, scrubbed and roughly chopped (not peeled)

2 celery stalks, roughly chopped, including leaves

1 medium onion, roughly chopped

1 (1-pound) package sliced button mushrooms

7 garlic cloves, smashed

3½ pounds beef soup bones (such as joints and knuckles; preferably from grass-fed beef)

2 bay leaves

2 fresh rosemary sprigs

2 teaspoons sea salt, or more as needed

2 tablespoons apple cider vinegar

2 quarts water

I have extolled the virtues of bone broth here and in my two other books, *The Hormone Fix* and *Keto-Green 16*. This is my favorite recipe for bone broth. You'll love it on this cleanse especially. It is also what I have when I go on my 3-day bone broth fasts.

Place the vegetables, garlic, soup bones, bay leaves, rosemary, salt, and vinegar in a large stockpot. Add the water and cover the pot. Bring to a boil over high heat, then reduce the heat to low and simmer for 12 hours. To make broth in a slow cooker, see page 228 of *The Hormone Fix*.

Use a spoon to carefully skim off any film on top of the broth. Pour the broth through a strainer and discard the solids. Taste the broth and add more salt as needed.

Variations: Substitute chicken, fish, or pork bones, or combine them all for one nutritious broth.

Opposite, left to right: Pork Bone Broth, page 240 • Roasted Chicken Bone Broth, page 241 • Dr. Anna's Beef Bone Broth, above

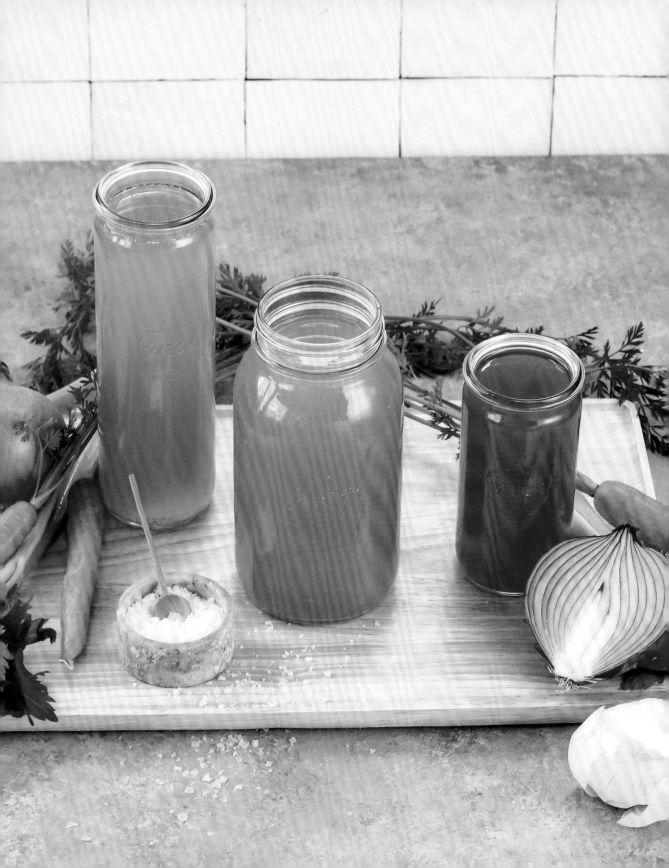

Dr. Anna's Mineral Broth   MAKES ABOUT 3 QUARTS

1 cup small cauliflower florets

1 cup broccoli slaw (or julienned stems from florets)

3 medium carrots, cut into thirds (unpeeled)

1 medium yellow onion or Vidalia, cut into chunks

1 leek (white and green parts), cut into thirds

1 bunch celery, including the heart and leaves, cut into quarters

4 garlic cloves, halved

½ bunch fresh parsley

3 bay leaves

3 to 4 quarts filtered water

1 teaspoon sea salt, or more as needed

For those of you who do not eat meat, this is the broth for you. And if you pause from meat during the year, this broth is ideal. It's highly alkalinizing and its vitamins, minerals, and antioxidants support great health at this time in our lives. Plus, it tastes so wonderful and can be used as a base for other vegan-style soups.

In a large stockpot, combine the vegetables, garlic, parsley, and bay leaves. Add 3 quarts of the water, cover the pot, and bring to a boil over high heat. Reduce the heat to low and simmer for about 2 hours (To make broth in a slow cooker, see page 228 of *The Hormone Fix*). As the broth simmers, some of the water will evaporate. Add more if the vegetables begin to peek out; they should remain covered.

Strain the broth through a large sieve or colander, then add the salt to taste. Let cool to room temperature, then refrigerate or freeze. (The broth can be stored in an airtight container in the refrigerator for 5 to 7 days or in the freezer for 4 months.)

Roasted-Garlic Bone Broth Soup
MAKES 6 TO 8 SERVINGS

2 tablespoons extra-virgin olive oil

1 medium onion, diced

1 (1-inch) piece fresh ginger, minced or finely chopped

4 fresh thyme sprigs

3 bay leaves

2 quarts Roasted Chicken Bone Broth (page 241) or bone broth of choice

6 garlic cloves

2 carrots, cut into 2-inch pieces (unpeeled)

2 celery stalks, cut into 2-inch pieces, with leaves

Sea salt and black pepper

½ cup chopped fresh parsley

There's lots of nutritional goodness in this broth, but let's zero in on the garlic. You've probably noticed that I use a lot of garlic in my recipes. There are many reasons, besides the fact that it tastes so good. The ancient Greek physician Hippocrates used to prescribe garlic to treat a variety of medical conditions. It has many healing properties: it can treat colds, reduce blood pressure, help the heart, detoxify the body, boost brain power, and possibly help us live longer. For all these reasons, I love garlic.

In a small skillet, heat the olive oil over medium heat. Add the onion and ginger, the thyme and bay leaves and sauté for about 5 minutes, until the onion is tender, stirring often.

Transfer the mixture to a large saucepan. Add the broth and garlic, giving it a quick stir. Bring to a boil over high heat, then cover, reduce the heat to low, and simmer for 20 minutes.

Remove the bay leaves and thyme sprigs. Pour into a blender (or use an immersion blender) and puree the broth until smooth.

Put the pureed broth back into the saucepan. Add the carrots, celery, and salt and pepper to taste. Cook until the vegetables are tender. Add the parsley at the very end, just before serving.

French-Onion Bone Broth Soup

MAKE 4 TO 6 SERVINGS

1 tablespoon butter or ghee (clarified butter)

1 tablespoon extra-virgin olive oil

4 large onions, thinly sliced

1 teaspoon garlic powder

2 teaspoons black pepper

1 quart beef, chicken, or vegetable broth, or bone broth

3 tablespoons Worcestershire sauce

Sea salt

I once had a batch of beef bone broth and wanted to do something different with it. I love French onion soup, and since I happened to have a bunch of onions in my fridge I put them to good use—with great results. You won't even miss the cheese or crusty bread usually served atop classic French onion soup!

In a large skillet, heat the butter and olive oil over medium heat. Add the onions, garlic powder, and pepper. Sauté for 10 to 15 minutes, until the onions are browned and caramelized.

Transfer the onions to a large saucepan. Add the broth, Worcestershire sauce, and salt to taste. Bring almost to a boil over high heat, then reduce the heat to low and simmer for at least 10 minutes or until onions are softened. Keep warm until ready to serve.

Mediterranean Lemon Soup

MAKES 6 TO 8 SERVINGS

3 pounds beef soup bones (preferably from grass-fed beef)

1 large onion, chopped

3 quarts water

2 cups frozen cauliflower rice

¼ cup chopped fresh parsley

¼ cup fresh lemon juice

Sea salt and black pepper

Ground cinnamon

Growing up, I had lemon soup with rice and meatballs every winter. There is no rice or meatballs here, but it's just as tasty. In fact, this soup is great on its own, or you can use it as a base to create heartier soups. The added cauliflower and parsley "soup up" its detoxifying benefits.

Place the bones and onion in a large stockpot. Add the water and cover the pot. Bring to a boil over high heat, then reduce the heat to low and simmer for 6 to 12 hours.

Strain the broth through a large, coarse-mesh sieve or colander. Add the cauliflower rice and parsley. Stir, then add the lemon juice and simmer for 5 more minutes. Season to taste with the salt and pepper, and garnish with a sprinkling of cinnamon.

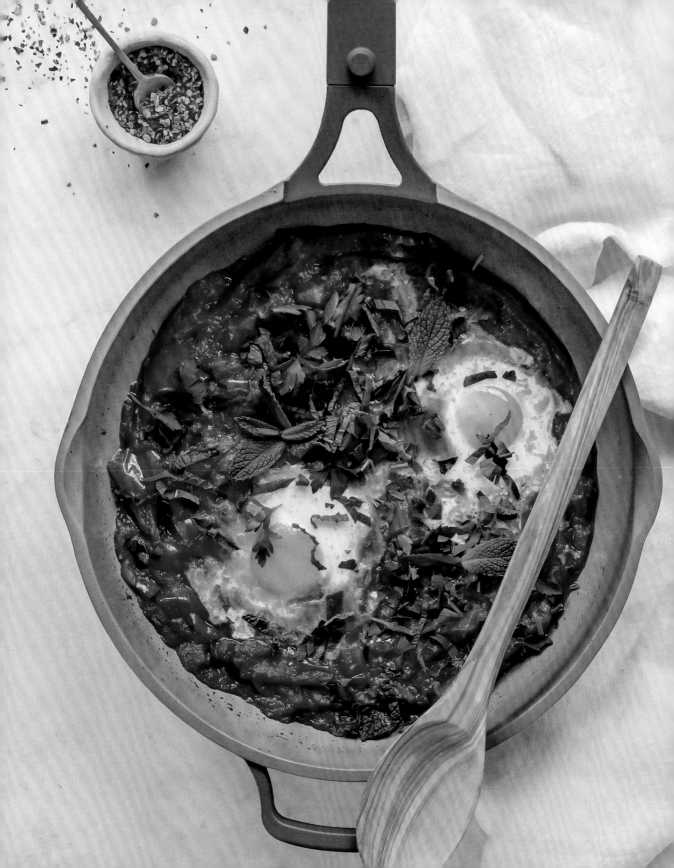

CHAPTER 13

The Carbohydrate Modification Plan Recipes

To view videos of some of the recipes in this plan, go to dranna.com/menupause-extras.

* These recipes can be used in other plans as well. See the recipe pages for more information.

Green Chia Pudding   MAKES 2 SERVINGS

4 tablespoons chia seeds

2 cups unsweetened
  almond milk

2 scoops Mighty Maca
  Plus, or 1 teaspoon
  maca root powder

1 teaspoon vanilla extract

½ cup fresh blueberries

½ cup avocado chunks

¼ cup sliced almonds

Accenting your diet with chia seeds is always a good idea. Indigenous to Mexico and Guatemala, these seeds were a staple for the ancient Aztecs and Mayans. In fact, *chia* is the ancient Mayan word for "strength." Within the tiny chia seed is a lot of fiber and omega-3 fatty acids, plenty of high-quality protein, and several essential minerals and antioxidants. Chia seeds are known to improve digestive health and lower risk factors for heart disease and diabetes. This recipe offers a yummy way to enjoy this powerhouse food. Just bear in mind that you need to soak the seeds for at least 2 hours before serving the pudding.

Put the chia seeds in the almond milk and stir 2 to 3 times during a 30-minute interval. Place in the refrigerator to chill for at least 2 hours, or overnight.

Pour the chia pudding into 2 serving bowls. Add the Mighty Maca and the vanilla and stir to blend in. Top each serving with some of the blueberries, avocado, and almonds.

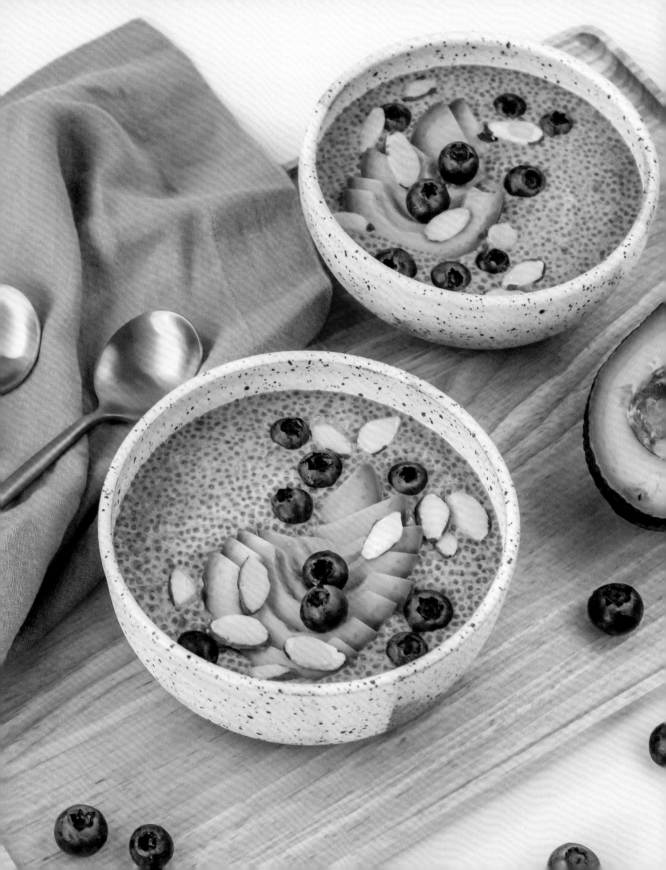

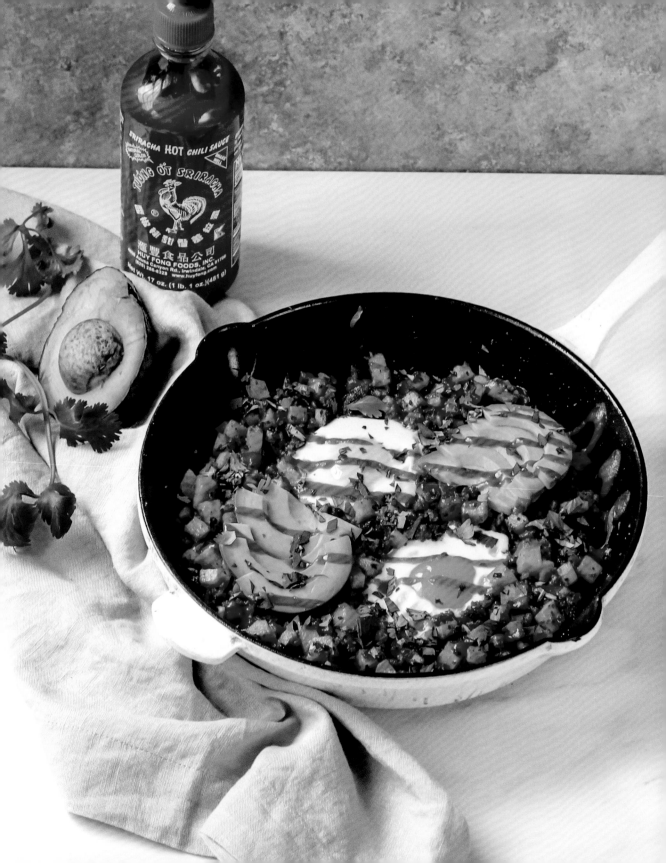

Texas Rodeo Breakfast Skillet MAKES 2 SERVINGS

8 ounces breakfast sausage meat

1 small sweet potato, peeled and diced

2 large eggs

4 slices of avocado

2 tablespoons chopped fresh cilantro

Sriracha or other hot sauce

I'm a big rodeo fan. My youngest daughter is a champion barrel racer, so I'm at rodeos a lot. Here's a hearty breakfast we often enjoy on weekends before heading off to our rodeos. It gives us the stamina and the nutrients to power through those days.

Preheat the oven to 400°F.

In a nonstick skillet, crumble in the sausage and brown for about 8 minutes over medium heat. With a slotted spoon, transfer the sausage to a paper towel–lined plate.

In the same skillet, add the sweet potato and cook for about 5 minutes over medium heat, until the pieces are crispy and cooked through. Return the sausage to the skillet and stir to combine.

Flatten the sausage mixture in the pan and use a wooden spoon to make 2 indentations, or "wells," in the mix. (If your skillet is not oven-safe, transfer the sausage mixture to a casserole dish first.) Crack the eggs into the wells.

Place the skillet in the oven and bake for 5 minutes, just long enough for the eggs to set. Switch the oven to broil and set to high heat. Slide the skillet under the broiler for a few minutes, but be careful not to let the yolks harden.

With a spatula, transfer the sausage-egg portions to serving plates. Top each with some avocado slices and sprinkle with cilantro. Serve with the Sriracha.

Bacon 'n' Egg Bundles MAKES 2 SERVINGS

6 strips no-sugar bacon

1 teaspoon butter or
   ghee (clarified butter)

2 large eggs

   Black pepper

Eggs and bacon—one of my favorite keto breakfasts. Here's a novel way to cook them. As you add the carbs, consider serving these eggs with a side of gluten-free oatmeal.

Preheat the oven to 325°F.

In a large skillet, cook the bacon over medium heat for about 8 minutes, until partially cooked but not yet crisp. Drain the bacon on a plate lined with paper towels.

Lightly grease 2 large muffin cups with the butter or ghee. Cut the bacon strips crosswise in half. Arrange 3 bacon halves in the bottom of each cup, then use the remaining bacon to line the sides of the muffin cups. Break an egg into each cup.

Bake for 12 to 18 minutes, until the egg whites are completely set and the yolks begin to thicken but are not hardened. Let cool slightly and then tip the egg bundles out of the muffin cups onto plates. Sprinkle with pepper and serve.

Baby Kale Breakfast Salad with Smoked Salmon and Avocado

MAKES 2 SERVINGS

2 teaspoons minced and mashed garlic

Sea salt

2 tablespoons extra-virgin olive oil

1 tablespoon red wine vinegar

Black pepper

6 cups lightly packed baby kale

6 ounces smoked salmon, cut into strips

½ firm ripe avocado, diced

2 tablespoons finely chopped red onion

2 teaspoons drained capers

Who said you can't have salad for breakfast? Yes, you can; it's one of the most delicious and nutritious ways to start your day. The centerpiece of this salad is smoked salmon, a breakfast favorite high in omega-3 fats, which help relieve menopausal depression.

Combine the garlic and 2 pinches of the salt in a medium bowl. Add the olive oil, vinegar, and pepper, and whisk to combine. Add the kale and toss to coat.

Place the kale salad on plates and top with the smoked salmon, avocado, and red onion. Sprinkle the capers over and enjoy.

NOTE: This recipe can be used on the Keto-Green Extreme Plan (without the black pepper) as a breakfast entree.

Shakshuka

1 tablespoon extra-virgin olive oil

¼ cup chopped onion

½ green bell pepper, cored and chopped

1 teaspoon minced garlic

¼ teaspoon ground coriander

¼ teaspoon paprika

⅛ teaspoon ground cumin

Pinch of red pepper flakes

Sea salt and black pepper

2 ripe large tomatoes, chopped

2 tablespoons tomato sauce

2 large eggs

1 tablespoon chopped fresh parsley

1 tablespoon chopped fresh mint

Never heard of shakshuka? I'm happy to introduce you. This is a yummy Middle Eastern breakfast that is both nutritious and filling. You'll love it! Plus, it contains certain spices—namely, cumin, fennel, coriander, and mint—that soothe digestive disorders like gas and bloating that can often crop up during menopause. This is optional, but you can serve this dish with your favorite bread.

Heat the olive oil in a medium skillet over medium-high heat. Add the onion, bell pepper, garlic, coriander, paprika, cumin, red pepper flakes, and salt and pepper to taste. Sauté, stirring occasionally, for about 5 minutes, until the vegetables have softened.

Add the fresh tomatoes and tomato sauce. Cover the skillet, lower the heat to medium, and let the mixture simmer for about 15 minutes. Uncover and cook a bit longer to allow the mixture to reduce and thicken a little.

With a wooden spoon, make 2 indentations, or "wells," in the tomato mixture. Gently crack an egg into each indention. Reduce the heat to low, cover the skillet, and cook for 2 to 3 minutes, until the egg whites are set but the yolks are still soft. Uncover and sprinkle on the parsley and mint before serving.

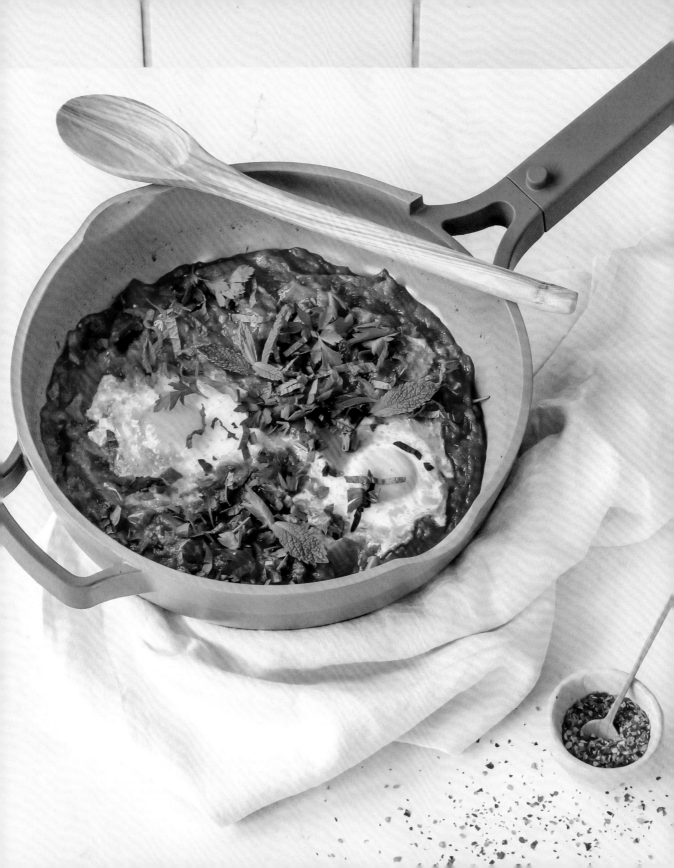

Poached Eggs on Swiss Chard

MAKES 2 SERVINGS

2 tablespoons extra-virgin olive oil, plus more for drizzling

4 garlic cloves, minced

1 pound rainbow Swiss chard, stems chopped fine and leaves cut into ½-inch-wide strips

1 teaspoon lemon pepper seasoning

¼ cup slivered almonds

½ lemon, cut into 2 wedges

2 large eggs, poached or fried, kept warm

It is okay—and indeed a great idea—to serve eggs on greens for breakfast. I love Swiss chard; it tastes like a milder version of spinach and it is so nutritious as an excellent source of vitamins K, A, and C, and the heart-healthy minerals magnesium, potassium, and iron. Here, I use both the leaves of the chard and the stems, which are often discarded.

Heat the olive oil in a medium skillet over medium heat. Add the garlic and cook for about 30 seconds, until fragrant. Stir in the chard and lemon pepper seasoning and increase the heat to medium-high. Cover and cook, stirring occasionally, for 2 to 3 minutes, until the chard is wilted and tender.

Stir the almonds into the chard, then divide the chard between 2 plates and squeeze a lemon wedge over each serving. Top each plate of chard with a cooked egg and drizzle with a little additional olive oil before serving.

Country Ham and White Bean Soup with Mustard Greens MAKES 2 SERVINGS

- 1 tablespoon extra-virgin olive oil
- 8 ounces sliced country ham, Canadian bacon, or other ham, trimmed of excess fat and diced
- ½ cup diced onion
- 1 teaspoon minced garlic
- 3 fresh thyme sprigs
- 1 (16-ounce) can Great Northern or cannellini beans, drained
- 2 cups chicken broth
- 1 (16-ounce) bag mustard greens, stemmed

  Sea salt and black pepper

I can't think of a more comforting soup than one made with country ham. Its smoky rich flavor blends well with the beans and mustard greens. This is a terrific one-pot meal with plenty of nourishment, alkalinity, and flavor.

In a large pot over medium heat, heat the olive oil. Add the ham and cook for 8 to 10 minutes, until it starts to brown. Use a slotted spoon to transfer the ham bits to a medium bowl.

Add the onion, garlic, and thyme to the pot. Stir well to combine, and sauté for 6 to 8 minutes, until translucent, but not browned. Add the beans and broth, then bring the liquid to a boil over medium-high heat. Reduce the heat to low and simmer for about 1 hour.

Add the ham and the mustard greens, and simmer for 6 to 8 minutes, until mustard greens are tender and wilted. Season to taste with salt and pepper, then serve.

Keto-Green Nachos MAKES 2 SERVINGS

For the faux-queso sauce

- ½ cup raw cashews
- ½ cup diced tomatoes with green chiles
- 2 tablespoons water
- 1 tablespoon lemon juice
- 1½ tablespoons nutritional yeast
- 1 teaspoon onion powder
- ½ teaspoon turmeric
- ½ teaspoon cumin
- ¼ teaspoon salt

For the nachos

- 2 tablespoons avocado oil or extra-virgin olive oil
- ½ cup chopped bell pepper (any color)
- 1 cup shredded cooked chicken breast meat
- 2 to 3 tablespoons salsa of choice
- 1 large zucchini, sliced into rounds
- 1 cup chopped greens (lettuce, spinach, kale, etc.)
- ½ medium cucumber, chopped
- 1 ripe medium tomato, chopped
- ½ cup prepared guacamole
- Fresh cilantro
- Lime wedges

This recipe has some tasty swaps that make it a delight to eat without the nutritional problems of the traditional. The cashews make the dairy-free faux-queso and tomato sauce, and zucchini rounds substitute for the otherwise high-carb chips. The key spice here is turmeric, a high-powered anti-inflammatory. Inflammation tends to increase during menopause, and turmeric can help reduce it.

Make the faux-queso. Place the cashews in a small saucepan and cover with water. Bring to boiling over high heat, then remove from the heat and cover the pan. Let sit for 15 minutes, then drain off the water and place the cashews in a blender.

Add the diced tomatoes with green chiles, water, lemon juice, nutritional yeast, onion powder, turmeric, cumin, and salt and blend until smooth. Add additional water to thin sauce if needed. Measure ½ to 1 cup of the cheese sauce for the nachos and store the remainder in a jar in the refrigerator.

Assemble the nachos. Heat 1 tablespoon of the avocado oil in a medium skillet over medium heat. Add the bell pepper and sauté for about 3 minutes, until the pepper begins to soften. Stir in the chicken and the salsa, and simmer until heated through. Transfer to a bowl and keep warm.

Add the remaining avocado oil to the skillet and place back over medium heat. Add the zucchini rounds and sauté for 3 minutes, until tender but still firm. Divide the rounds between 2 plates. Top with the chicken mixture.

Heat the queso sauce in a small saucepan over medium heat, and then spoon over the nachos. Top with the chopped greens, cucumber, tomato, and guacamole. Also, garnish with fresh cilantro and lime wedges before serving. Serve at once.

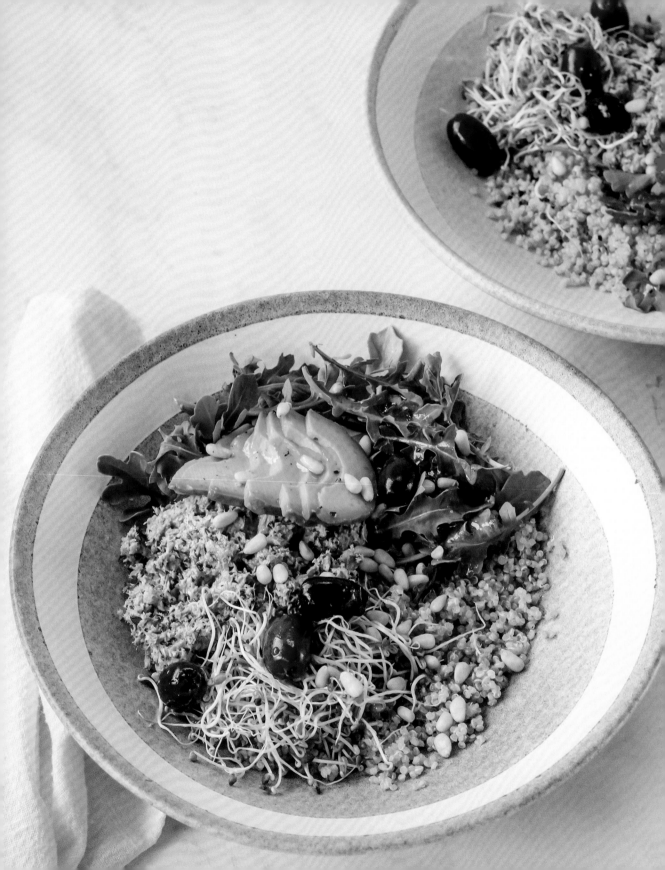

Salmon Quinoa Bowl MAKES 2 SERVINGS

1 (6-ounce) can salmon, preferably wild-caught

1½ tablespoons Vegenaise

¼ cup chopped fresh cilantro

1 teaspoon ground cumin

2 tablespoons extra-virgin olive oil

Juice of 1 lemon

¼ teaspoon black pepper

1 cup cooked quinoa (follow directions on package)

½ cup diced avocado

⅓ cup bean sprouts of choice

¼ cup pine nuts

1 cup chopped fresh arugula

8 pitted Kalamata olives

Bowl meals like this are not only easy to make but also convenient because you can wrap and take them to work. One of the key ingredients here is quinoa, a grain-like superfood that is high in protein.

In a small bowl, mix the salmon, Vegenaise, cilantro, and cumin.

In another small bowl, combine the olive oil, lemon juice, and black pepper to taste.

Divide the quinoa between 2 serving bowls. Place half the salmon mixture in each bowl atop the quinoa. Sprinkle the bowls with the avocado, sprouts, pine nuts, arugula, and olives. Drizzle with the oil and lemon mixture, and serve.

Tarragon Chicken Salad with Apples and Pecans

MAKES 2 SERVINGS

2 tablespoons sea salt

2 cups water

2 (6- to 8-ounce) boneless, skinless chicken breasts

¼ cup Vegenaise

2 teaspoons dried tarragon

1 small apple, peeled, cored, and diced (about ¾ cup)

1 teaspoon grated lemon zest

Juice of 1 lemon

¼ cup toasted chopped pecans

¼ teaspoon black pepper

Tarragon lends a delicate licorice edge to dishes. It also has some surprising health benefits. One such benefit is that it may decrease blood sugar and increase insulin sensitivity. That's important during menopause, since insulin problems can cause hot flashes.

Dissolve 1 tablespoon of the salt in 1 cup of the water. Place the chicken breasts in the brine to soak for 15 to 30 minutes.

Add the remaining cup water and remaining tablespoon salt in a medium skillet with high sides. Bring the water to a low simmer.

Remove the chicken from the brine, pat dry, then add to the simmering water. If not submerged, add a bit more water to cover. Put the lid on the skillet and simmer over low heat for 15 to 20 minutes, until chicken is cooked through. Check for doneness by cutting into a breast; it should not have any pinkness. Transfer the chicken to a plate to cool.

Chop the chicken into small pieces, discarding any fat or tendon.

In a medium bowl, combine the Vegenaise, tarragon, apple, lemon zest, lemon juice, pecans, and pepper. Add the chicken, stir to combine, and chill for 30 minutes before serving.

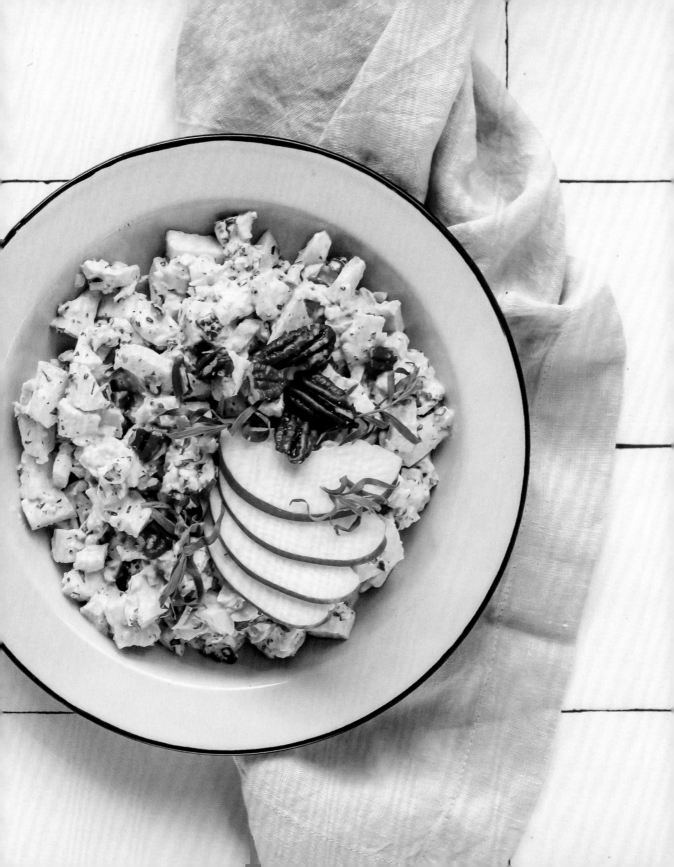

Twice-Baked Sweet Potatoes

MAKES 2 SERVINGS

2 medium sweet potatoes

4 teaspoons butter or ghee (clarified butter)

2 tablespoons pure maple syrup

1 teaspoon vanilla extract

4 tablespoons chopped pecans

1 tablespoon coconut sugar

Sweet potatoes are my favorite carb. They are yummy by themselves, or you can dress them up, as in this recipe. They are full of vitamins, fiber, and minerals. Plus, unlike white potatoes, they are digested slowly, so they have minimal impact on your blood sugar levels. And don't forget that the vitamin A they contain is beneficial for vaginal lubrication. They also help with a good night's sleep.

Preheat the oven to 350°F.

Wrap the sweet potatoes in aluminum foil and bake for 1 hour, until soft. Remove the sweet potatoes but leave the oven turned on.

Let the sweet potatoes cool slightly, then remove the alumnium foil. Cut them in half lengthwise and scoop out the flesh into a small bowl. Add 2 teaspoons of the butter, the maple syrup, and vanilla. Mash well, then spoon the mixture into the potato skins.

Melt the remaining 2 teaspoons butter in a small saucepan or the microwave. In a small bowl, combine the pecans, coconut sugar, and the melted butter. Top the stuffed potatoes with this mixture. Return the sweet potatoes to the oven for 5 minutes, until heated through.

Brussels Me Up Salad

MAKES 2 SERVINGS

Here is another pairing of Brussel sprouts and radishes, this time in a delicious salad along with the super-food kale. This is one salad that will really give you a nutrient boost. Brussels sprouts, radishes, and kale are important detoxifying vegetables that help get rid of excess and harmful estrogens in your body for better hormonal balance.

1 cup shredded Brussels sprouts

1 cup shredded stemmed kale

¼ cup chopped onion

2 tablespoons chopped almonds

2 radishes, thinly sliced

2 to 3 tablespoons extra-virgin olive oil

1 to 2 tablespoons no-sugar balsamic vinegar

Sea salt and black pepper

Combine the sprouts, kale, onion, almonds, and radishes in a medium bowl. Add the olive oil and vinegar and toss well. Season to taste with salt and pepper.

NOTE: This recipe can be used on the Keto-Green Plant-Based Detox Plan.

Anytime Keto-Green Salad

MAKES 2 SERVINGS

This recipe is DIY. I've listed the best salad ingredients for you. Now, all you have to do is select the ones you like best, in the desired amounts, and you're good to go. The greens and nuts are hormone balancing, and the protein provides fat-burning power.

Large handful of mixed baby greens, fresh spinach, or kale

Sliced ripe tomatoes

Cucumber slices

Bean sprouts

Sunflower seeds

Slivered almonds

Poached salmon or chicken, canned tuna or sardines, hard-boiled eggs, or other protein choice

Extra-virgin olive oil

Vinegar of choice

In a medium bowl, toss together the greens, tomato, and cucumber and place on plates. Top with the sprouts, sunflower seeds, and/or slivered almonds. Arrange your choice of protein on top, then drizzle a little olive oil and vinegar over the top.

Wild Rice Pilaf MAKES 2 TO 3 SERVINGS

- ½ **cup wild rice**
- ½ **cup long-grain brown rice**
- 2 **teaspoons coconut oil**
- ¼ **cup finely diced onion**
- ¼ **cup finely diced celery**
- ¼ **cup grated carrot**
- ¼ **cup diced fresh mushrooms (optional)**
- ¼ **cup roughly chopped pecans or slivered almonds (optional)**
- ¼ **teaspoon each ground thyme, rosemary, and sage**
- ½ **teaspoon sea salt**
- ½ **teaspoon black pepper**
- 2 **cups chicken broth**

This is a lovely side dish and the source of good-guy carbs—wild rice and brown rice— both high in fiber, B vitamins, and of course flavor. Added to the mix are mushrooms (always delicious with rice), vitamin A-rich carrots, fiber-loaded celery, and alkaline herbs. All these ingredients are typical additions to rice pilaf. Note: you can use cauliflower rice if you want to keep your carbohydrates lower.

In separate bowls, combine the wild rice and brown rice with water to cover. Allow to soak for 4 hours or overnight. Rinse the rice after soaking.

Heat the coconut oil in a medium pot over medium-high heat. Add the onion, celery, carrot, mushrooms, and pecans, then sprinkle with the thyme, rosemary, and sage. Add the salt and pepper and sauté for about 5 minutes, until the vegetables are starting to soften.

Add both rices and stir well for an additional minute. Then add the broth and bring to a boil. Stir, reduce the heat to low, cover, and simmer for about 50 minutes, until both types of rice are cooked. Fluff with a fork and serve.

Pan-Seared Coriander Lamb Chops MAKES 2 SERVINGS

6 lamb rib chops

1 tablespoon coriander seeds (or ground coriander)

2 teaspoons sea salt

2 teaspoons black peppercorns (or ground black pepper)

1 tablespoon extra-virgin olive oil

Here is an amazingly easy way to fix lamb chops: simply sear them in a skillet with a few spices. Taking center stage here are coriander seeds, which increase the metabolism, regulate blood sugar, and improve immune function. Simple, but how does it taste? Sharp but sweet—perfect for lamb chops.

About 1 hour before cooking, allow the chops to come to room temperature.

With a mortar and pestle, or spice grinder, combine and grind together the coriander seeds, salt, and peppercorns. Spread the chops on both sides with the spice mixture.

Put the olive oil in a medium cast-iron skillet over medium-high heat. Let it get very hot, but not smoking, then add the chops. Sauté for about 2 minutes on each side for medium rare or for 3 to 4 minutes on each side for well done, allowing a nice crust to form on each side. Remove from the skillet and let rest for 5 minutes. Transfer the chops to plates and pour the pan juices over, then serve.

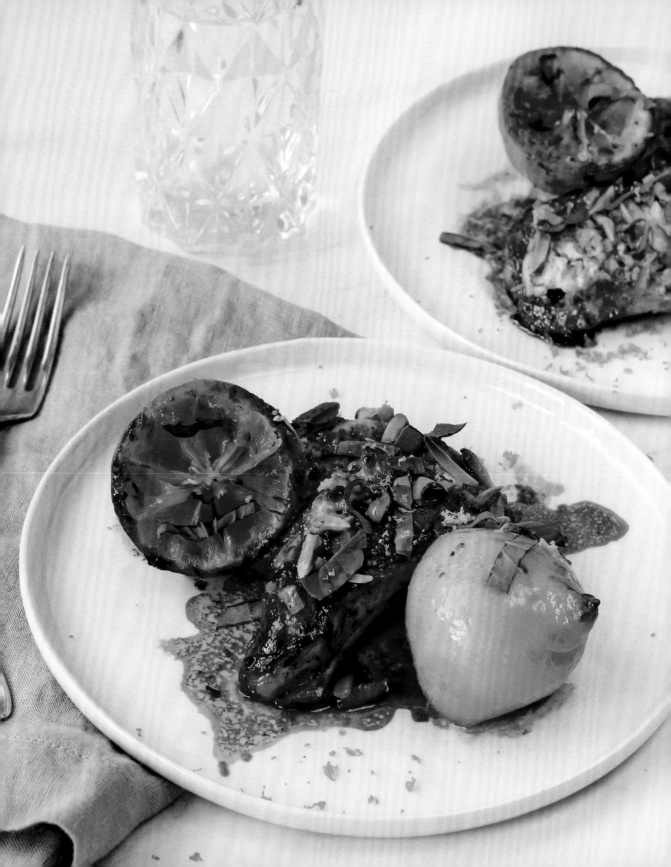

Chicken with Goat Cheese, Fig Jam, and Basil

MAKES 2 SERVINGS

2 chicken cutlets, 4 to 6 ounces each

1 teaspoon sea salt

1 teaspoon black pepper

1 teaspoon minced fresh rosemary

1 tablespoon butter or ghee (clarified butter)

1 tablespoon extra-virgin olive oil

1 (8-ounce) jar Adriatic fig spread (or apricot or raspberry jam)

1 (4-ounce) log goat cheese (chèvre; see Note)

¼ cup slivered almonds

½ cup dry white wine

2 lemons, cut in half

¼ cup fresh basil leaves, julienned

Grated zest from 2 lemons

NOTE: Omit the goat cheese if you're dairy-free.

Figs have been called the "food of the gods," and for good reason. They are juicy, delicious, and full of fiber. This recipe blends alkaline herbs, protein-rich almonds, and a little dairy in the form of goat cheese. Goat cheese is easier to digest than cow's or sheep's milk cheeses. Plus, it supplies gut-friendly probiotics. You won't use all the fig jam or the chèvre in the recipe, but that's reason enough to make this another time!

Preheat the oven to 425°F. Place the rack close to the oven top.

Heat a large oven-proof skillet over low. (If you don't have an oven-proof skillet, transfer the chicken mixture into a casserole dish before placing in the oven.)

Season both sides of the cutlets with salt, pepper, and rosemary. Add the olive oil and butter to the skillet and heat until sizzling but not smoking. Add the chicken cutlets and sauté about 3 minutes per side, until browned.

Top the cutlets with 1 or 2 tablespoons of the fig spread, 1 to 2 tablespoons of goat cheese, and 1 to 2 tablespoons of the almonds.

Add the wine to the skillet and place the lemon halves alongside the cutlets. Transfer the skillet to the oven and bake 7 to 10 minutes, until the cheese is melted and the chicken is cooked through.

Transfer the cutlets to plates and garnish with the basil and lemon zest. Serve with the roasted lemon halves on the side.

Za'atar-Roasted Salmon with Garlicky Bean Mash MAKES 2 SERVINGS

2 salmon fillets, 4 to 6 ounces each (preferably wild-caught)

2 tablespoons extra-virgin olive oil

Sea salt and black pepper

3 tablespoons za'atar

2 tablespoons butter or ghee

1 garlic clove, crushed

Grated zest of 1 lemon

1 (16-ounce) can kidney beans, drained and rinsed

2 tablespoons water, or more as needed

1 lemon, cut into wedges

I use za'atar frequently in my cooking. This Middle Eastern spice mix commonly contains dried thyme, oregano, sumac, and sesame seeds. All these spices contain phytonutrients that are valuable for hormonal harmony. This dish is earthy, nutty, zesty, and tangy.

Preheat the oven to 400°F.

Place the salmon fillets on a baking sheet, skin side down. Drizzle evenly with the olive oil and season with ½ teaspoon each of the salt and pepper. Sprinkle the za'atar over the fish, coating as much of the surface as you can. Place the fish into the oven and bake for 11 to 13 minutes, until the fillets are just cooked through.

Meanwhile, melt the butter in a medium skillet over low heat. Sauté the garlic and lemon zest for a few minutes. Add the beans, water, ½ teaspoon salt, and ¼ teaspoon pepper. Heat and stir until the beans are warmed through. Then use a fork or potato masher to mash them in the pan. If the mixture looks dry, add a bit more water.

Spread the bean mixture on serving plates. Lay the fish fillets on top, and serve with lemon wedges.

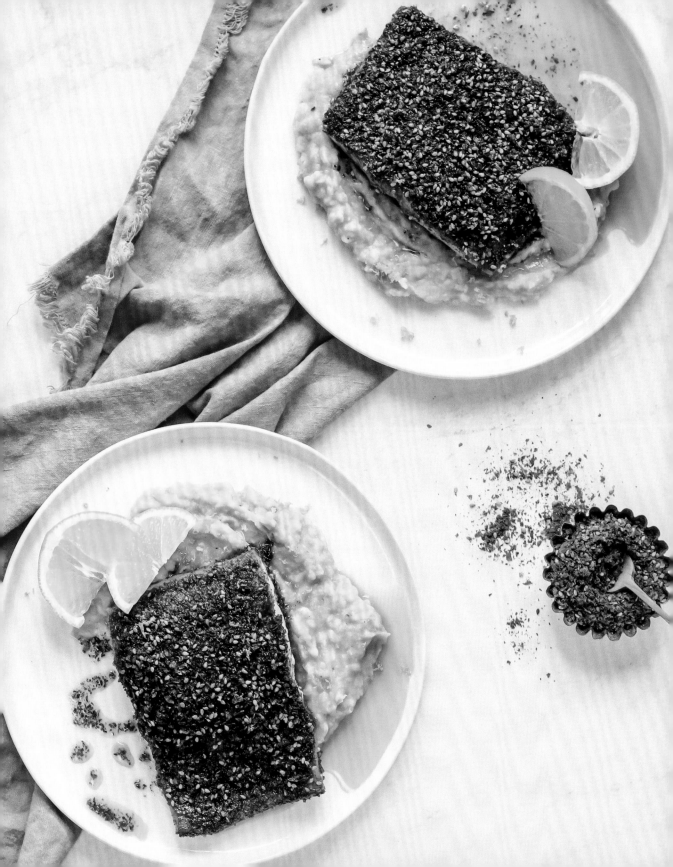

Country Ranch Turkey Meatloaf

MAKES 6 SERVINGS

For the meatloaf

- 2 tablespoons butter or ghee (clarified butter)
- 1 small onion, minced
- 1 to 2 garlic cloves, minced
- 2 large handfuls chopped fresh spinach
- Sea salt and black pepper
- 1½ pounds ground turkey (moderately lean)
- 2 large eggs
- ¼ cup almond flour
- ½ teaspoon onion powder
- ½ teaspoon garlic powder
- ½ teaspoon paprika
- 1 tablespoon spicy brown mustard

For the ranch sauce

- ½ cup Vegenaise or mayonnaise
- 3 tablespoons coconut cream
- ½ teaspoon garlic powder
- ½ teaspoon onion powder
- 2 teaspoons dried chives
- ¼ teaspoon dried dill
- 1 teaspoon fresh lemon juice
- ⅛ to ¼ teaspoon sea salt, or more as needed

I love to make meatloaf because it is both forgiving and versatile. Many times, I use whatever I have on hand, while always giving it a healthy twist. This recipe is a good example of that. It sneaks in the spinach, just in case you have some veggie haters in your family. I use almond flour here as the binder to keep the recipe gluten-free and easy on digestion. Leftovers will keep in the fridge for three days, well wrapped.

Make the meatloaf. Preheat the oven to 350°F. Use a bit of the butter to very lightly grease a 9-by-5-inch loaf pan.

Heat the remaining butter in a large skillet over medium heat. Add the onion and garlic and sauté for 3 minutes, until translucent. Add the spinach and cook for about 5 minutes, until wilted. Sprinkle with a bit of salt. Let cool to room temperature.

In a large bowl, combine the turkey, eggs, almond flour, ¾ teaspoon salt, ⅛ teaspoon pepper, onion and garlic powders, paprika, and mustard. Stir and add the spinach mixture.

Place the meat mixture in the loaf pan, shaping to fill the pan but rounding the top a bit. Bake for 45 to 50 minutes, until done in the center (no longer pink and juices run clear). Let the meatloaf rest for about 10 minutes.

Make the ranch sauce: Whisk together the ranch sauce ingredients.

When ready to serve, slice the meatloaf in the pan. Spoon the sauce over the slices and serve.

Coriander-Garlic Shrimp

MAKES 2 SERVINGS

For the spice mix

- 1½ cups chopped fresh cilantro
- 4 to 5 garlic cloves
- 1 (¼-inch) piece fresh ginger
- 1 serrano pepper
- 1 teaspoon ground cumin
- 1 teaspoon ground coriander
- 1 teaspoon ground turmeric
- ½ teaspoon black pepper
  - Sea salt

For the shrimp

- 1 tablespoon butter or ghee (clarified butter)
- 1 medium onion, finely chopped
- 1½ teaspoons almond flour
- 1 cup water
- 2 small ripe tomatoes, chopped
- 2 cups chopped fresh spinach
- 2 cups chopped fresh kale
- 7 ounces peeled and deveined shrimp (any size)

Here is another of my favorite shrimp dishes. It has a lot of scrumptious ingredients, but it doesn't take long to prepare. The herbs and veggies are highly alkaline, and your body will love you for them. Serve this with cauliflower rice, brown rice, or quinoa.

Make the spice mix. Combine the ingredients in a blender and blend well.

Make the shrimp. Heat the butter in a large skillet over medium heat. Add the onion and sauté for 3 minutes, until translucent. Add the spice mixture and cook until fragrant, stirring often.

Add the almond flour, water, tomatoes, spinach, kale, and shrimp. Cook for about 5 minutes, until the greens are wilted and the shrimp are opaque. Serve.

Gluten-Free Chocolate Chip Cookies

MAKES ABOUT 2 DOZEN

2½ **cups almond flour**

¼ **teaspoon sea salt**

¼ **teaspoon baking soda**

1 **cup stevia dark chocolate chips**

2 **large eggs**

½ **cup (1 stick) butter, melted and slightly cooled**

1 **tablespoon vanilla extract**

½ **cup raw honey or coconut nectar**

Talk about comfort foods! Chocolate chip cookies spell comfort with a capital "C." Part of the comfort is the aroma you have when you pull them out of the oven. Using stevia-sweetened chocolate chips helps downsize the sugar content.

Preheat the oven to 350°F. Line a baking sheet with parchment paper.

In a large bowl, combine the almond flour, salt, baking soda, and chocolate chips.

In a small bowl, combine the eggs, melted butter, vanilla, and honey. Add the wet ingredients to the dry ingredients and stir to mix well.

Form the dough into 1-inch balls and transfer the balls to the baking sheet, leaving a 1-inch space between them. Press the balls slightly to flatten. Bake for 15 to 17 minutes, until the cookies are firm. Let cool briefly on the baking sheet and then transfer to a rack to cool completely.

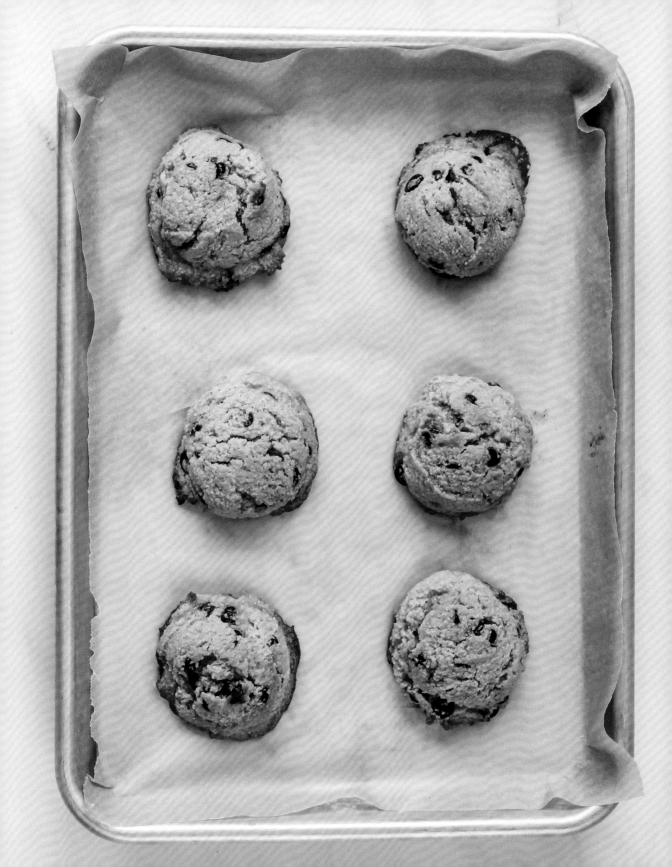

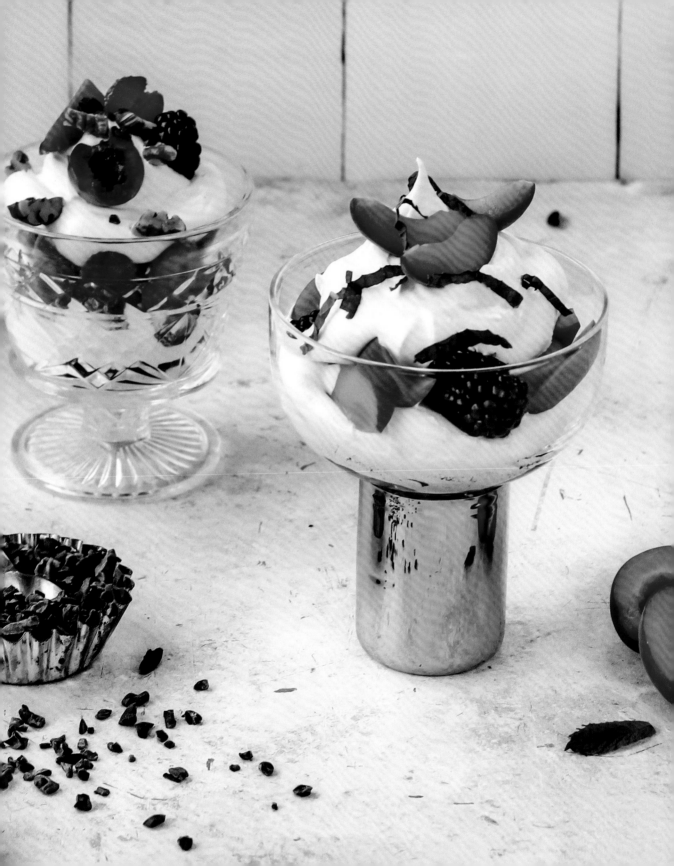

DIY Summer Fruit Parfait
MAKES 2 SERVINGS

This parfait gives you the freedom to choose the fruits and toppings you love. Experiment and find just the right combination for your palate. Go high on the berries, though, because they are powerful fighters against inflammation, which tends to increase during menopause.

2 cups mixed fruit: blueberries, strawberries, raspberries, blackberries, sliced peaches, and sliced plums

Coconut cream whip (from an 8-ounce carton)

Chopped nuts

Cacao nibs

Unsweetened shredded coconut

Chopped fresh mint or basil

In 2 dessert bowls, alternate layers of the fruit with some whipped coconut cream, nuts, cacao nibs, and coconut. Garnish with the mint or basil.

Chocolaty Freezer Fudge
MAKES 12 TO 16 PIECES

This fat-boosting, hunger-busting recipe is a take on the fat bomb but made as a fudge instead. This is so easy to make, which explains why I have some in my freezer at all times.

¾ cup almond butter

¾ cup cashew butter

⅓ cup coconut oil, softened

5 tablespoons organic unsweetened cacao powder

30 drops stevia, or more as needed

1 teaspoon vanilla extract

Pinch of sea salt

Place the almond butter, cashew butter, coconut oil, cacao powder, stevia, vanilla, and salt in a medium bowl. Using a hand mixer, beat together to form a thick, uniform paste.

Line a large plate or small baking sheet with parchment paper. Spread the fudge evenly over the paper. Place the fudge in the freezer to chill for about 30 minutes. Cut into pieces or store in the freezer whole and break off small squares to enjoy.

Lemon Panna Cotta MAKES 8 SERVINGS

1 cup unsweetened almond milk

1 packet unflavored gelatin

3 cups coconut cream

1 (2-inch) piece of vanilla bean, split lengthwise, or 2 teaspoons vanilla extract

2 teaspoons grated lemon zest

6 tablespoons organic cane sugar or honey

Pinch of sea salt

¼ cup fresh lemon juice

Panna cotta is Italian for "cooked cream," and that's exactly what this is: a dessert of sweetened coconut cream that is thickened with gelatin and molded. This version has a lemony flavor that is a delight to the taste buds. I love to cook with coconut cream; it is rich and creamy, but also contains a fatty acid called monolaurin that can kill harmful microorganisms. If desired, top the panna cotta with sliced fresh fruit, coconut flakes, or more lemon zest.

Pour the almond milk into a medium saucepan and sprinkle the surface evenly with the gelatin. Let stand 10 minutes, to soften.

Pour the coconut cream into a large pitcher. Use a paring knife to scrape the vanilla seeds into the cream, then add the bean. Add the lemon zest and gently stir.

Arrange 8 (4-ounce) ramekins on a baking sheet.

Heat the milk and gelatin mixture over high heat, stirring constantly, until the gelatin is dissolved, about 1½ minutes. Remove the saucepan from the heat and add the sugar and salt; stir until dissolved, about 1 minute. Then slowly pour the cream mixture into the saucepan, stirring constantly. Strain the cream mixture back into the pitcher, discard the vanilla bean, and stir in the lemon juice. Pour the mixture into the ramekins.

Cover the baking sheet with plastic wrap, making sure that the plastic does not touch the fillings in the ramekins. Refrigerate until just set, about 4 hours.

Riesling Poached Pears MAKES 2 SERVINGS

1 cup Riesling or other fruity white wine

¼ cup organic cane sugar

1 vanilla bean

1 cinnamon stick

2 whole cloves

Peel of 1 navel orange

2 firm pears

Coconut cream whip (from 8-ounce carton; optional)

Said W. C. Fields: "I cook with wine, sometimes I even add it to the food." Here's a recipe in which you definitely want to add the wine—as a poaching liquid. I love to eat pears raw, but they're also fun to poach for a tasty, nutritious dessert. Pears are also one of the most fiber-rich foods you can eat to support regularity. This recipe can be whipped up in no time.

Place the wine, sugar, vanilla bean, cinnamon stick, cloves, and orange peel in a medium pot and bring to a boil. Stir to dissolve the sugar and reduce the heat to low.

Peel the pears and slice in half lengthwise. Remove the core and seeds, then gently drop them into the simmering liquid. (If they are not fully covered, add more wine to cover them.) Poach for about 10 minutes if you have ripe pears, 20 minutes for almost ripe pears, and 35 minutes for totally unripe pears. Test for doneness by piercing one pear with the pointed end of a sharp knife. It should be just soft but not mushy.

Carefully remove the pears with a slotted spoon and place 2 halves in each serving dish. Cover with foil to keep warm.

Simmer the poaching liquid for 5 to 7 minutes, until reduced to a syrup-like consistency. Strain through a fine-mesh strainer and discard the solids. Drizzle the pears with the syrup and top with the coconut cream, if desired.

Vanilla and Fig Scones with Pistachios

MAKES 6 TO 8 SCONES

2½ cups almond flour

½ teaspoon sea salt

½ teaspoon baking soda

⅓ cup coconut oil, melted

¼ cup honey

2 large eggs

1 teaspoon vanilla extract

½ cup chopped dried figs, plus some for garnish

½ cup roughly chopped pistachios

For a great dessert or breakfast, you can't go wrong with a scone. A scone is a baked good, usually made with wheat flour and butter. I use almond flour instead to reduce the carbs and increase the nutrition. The pastry has been enjoyed in Scotland since 1513, and its name probably derives from the Dutch word for "bread." I add figs and pistachios here to sweeten the scones and give them a bit of crunch.

Preheat the oven to 350°F. Line a large baking sheet with parchment paper.

In a large bowl, combine the almond flour, salt, and baking soda.

In a medium bowl, whisk together the oil, honey, eggs, and vanilla. Stir the wet ingredients into the dry until thoroughly combined. Fold in the ½ cup of figs and the pistachios.

Place the dough on the baking sheet and shape into a rectangle about 1 inch thick. Cut into squares and then cut the squares diagonally into triangular wedges. Separate the wedges so they are about 1 inch apart to allow for even cooking. Press a few pieces of fig into the top of each wedge.

Bake for 12 to 17 minutes, until golden brown and a toothpick inserted in a scone comes out clean. Let cool for 30 minutes on the baking sheet, then serve.

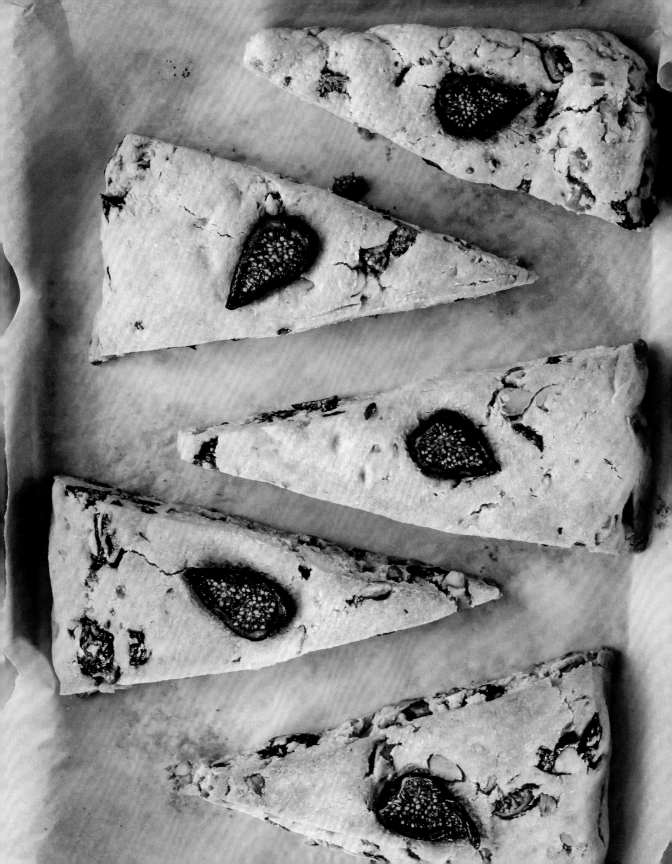

Keto Almond Delight MAKES 14 TO 16 BARS

For the bars

- 2 cups unsweetened shredded coconut
- ½ cup full-fat coconut milk
- ½ teaspoon almond extract
- Pinch of sea salt
- ¾ cup coconut oil
- ½ vanilla bean, split and seeds scraped out
- 2 tablespoons erythritol (optional)
- 14 to 16 whole almonds

For the topping and chocolate coating

- 1 cup 100% or 85% cacao chocolate chips
- 2 teaspoons coconut oil

Can you eat candy bars while still eating healthfully? You bet you can, and this recipe is a great example. Candy bars are usually sugar disasters, but this one swaps the sugar for erythritol, a tasty zero-calorie sweetener. The almondy-coconutty-chocolaty flavor is happiness the moment the bar touches your lips. Enjoy these when you get cravings or hunger pangs; the healthy fat will zap those in no time.

Make the bars. Place the coconut into the bowl of a food processor and process to form smaller crumbs. Add the coconut milk, almond extract, salt, coconut oil, vanilla bean, and sweetener (if using). Process until well combined.

Place a large piece of parchment paper on your counter, and spoon the coconut mixture across the sheet, forming a strip about 12 inches long. Don't go all the way to the edges of the paper. Bring up one long side of the paper and use it to begin rolling the strip, folding tightly. Using your fingers, smooth the log to remove any air pockets and make it even. Carefully place the wrapped log on a sheet pan and freeze for about 30 minutes, until firm enough to slice. (Alternatively, I have used a mini-cookie scoop to lay out the dough in portions on the parchment-lined sheet pan.)

Remove the coconut log from the freezer and let sit a few minutes on the counter. Transfer the log to the counter and line the sheet pan with parchment paper.

Using a very sharp knife, slice the log into ¾-inch-thick bars and place the bars on the sheet pan. Press an almond lightly into each bar. Place the sheet pan in the refrigerator to chill for 30 minutes to firm up again.

Make the coating. Melt the chocolate chips and coconut oil carefully in a double boiler.

Remove the bars from the refrigerator and carefully dip each into the warm chocolate mixture. (Alternatively, you could spoon the chocolate over the tops to have the coating only on the top and sides. Whatever feels more fun to you!) Let cool again, then store the bars in an airtight container in the refrigerator for up to 1 week or freeze for up to 3 months.

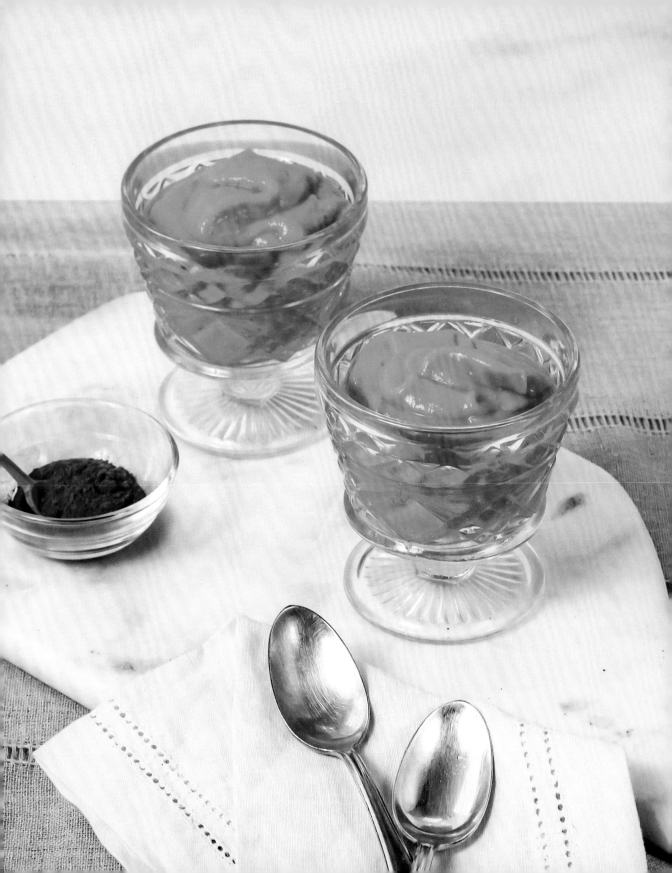

Pumpkin Mango Mousse

MAKES 2 SERVINGS

1 cup canned pumpkin puree

12 to 20 small chunks of frozen mango

½ cup coconut yogurt

Ground nutmeg, cinnamon, or cardamom

Mango is a tropical fruit I often recommend for digestive purposes. It contains a group of digestive enzymes called amylases, which break down carbs from starch into sugars like glucose and maltose for better absorption. From a flavor standpoint, mango and pumpkin are the perfect taste couple—very rich, fruity, and naturally sweet.

Blend the pumpkin, mango, and yogurt in a blender. Flavor with the spices and serve in parfait glasses.

CHAPTER 14

Pause What No Longer Serves You

You have learned to pause certain foods on this program to help you through menopause. You have tuned in to how these pauses make you feel. You know how your body responds after you make necessary nutritional changes.

Congratulations are in order! I'm thrilled you have come this far, and that you now have essential tools and knowledge to help you along your journey ahead.

There is more to talk about, however. It is also important to pause, or even eliminate, other habits and situations to help you get through this time in your life. Nothing is more painful, draining, or health limiting than being stuck in a habit that does not serve you well. Not only does it drain your energy, but it also keeps you from achieving happiness and health and becoming all you were meant to be. Inactivity, smoking, stress, and negative thinking—these are examples of things that do not serve us or our well-being. To be our best selves right now and in the future, some things need to go!

Here's another way to look at this. When I was a little girl, my favorite toy was a Barbie townhouse. It had three stories, was pink, with very cool furniture. But as I got older, that toy no longer served me in the same way it as did when I was a child. I had to let it go.

What else do we need to let go, besides poor nutritional habits? There are five other things that will stand in your way of a positive transition through menopause to an awesome life beyond. Take inventory and see if any of these exist in your life right now.

Inactivity

If you're not exercising, you're doing your hormones a disservice, especially your three master hormones—insulin, cortisol, and oxytocin. Exercise, for example, makes muscle cells use insulin more effectively. Working out is a great way to prevent insulin resistance—and the hot flashes it triggers! Exercise can also drive away excess cortisol in your body, brought on by chronic stress. And, the hormone of love and bonding, oxytocin, increases when you exercise—one of the reasons you feel so great after a workout.

To be honest, I've paused exercise at times in my life, but with negative consequences like poor weight control and irritability. I'm not someone who has made exercise a priority because I love it. Oh, no. It is a necessity, and I'm always happy after the deed has been done. I much prefer to curl up with a good book. So, creating more ways to be active has been essential to my Keto-Green way of life—which is why I purchased a treadmill desk. When I prioritize workouts, I feel better and I have more energy. Tip: Encourage yourself as I do with my mantra: "I will be so happy when I am done!"

As for how to exercise, your options are endless. Aerobic activities, such as walking, jogging, swimming, biking, and dancing help raise HDL cholesterol levels, the "good" cholesterol. Weight-bearing exercises help increase bone mass. And exercise, in general, help improve mood by elevating other hormones called endorphins. These also help the body fight stress.

Exercise doesn't mean you have to start running marathons, so if you have paused exercise in the past, there are still activities you can participate in. Low-impact activities like yoga, swimming, and walking are all beneficial forms of exercise. Strength training keeps muscles strong and helps burn fat, while stretching helps improve flexibility. Whatever you choose, just try to move!

Unhealthy Substances

These include any habit that is physically harmful to your health, such as smoking, drugs, and excessive drinking. These not only endanger health but they also, in the long term, can lead to chronic diseases. These habits need to be not just paused but also let go of completely.

For habit change, here is something I've found very effective in helping me deal differently with circumstances that previously caused me to respond with a "habit" that wasn't useful: *take the next right step.*

Ask yourself: What is the one next right step I can take today toward my purpose, goals, commitments, relationships, and other life-fortifying pursuits? Prioritize and do just the one next right step. Doing this keeps me in forward motion and away from past traumas, pain, and stress. God gave us eyes in front, on our face, to look forward not back, as I like to say.

Based on what you know to be your next right step, you have an opportunity to make a different decision *today*! Choose now to do something differently.

Stress

When we are under stress, our body goes into a state of "fight, flight, or freeze." That means that we don't focus on ourselves in a healthy way. We don't eat right or get enough sleep. We don't concentrate on our relationships with our families and children.

We don't have the energy to support our friends and community. We just can't cope, bond, or be in the moment for anyone. And we fail to say no to that emotional eating!

In the absence of chronic stress, however, we thrive. Our behavioral and relationship tendencies are positive and nurturing. We "feed and breed," meaning we bond with and nurture our family and children. We "tend and befriend" in order to nurture and support our community and friends. And we "rest and digest," taking care of our basic needs for good food, healthy lifestyle habits, and adequate rest.

For these reasons, we absolutely need lifestyle upgrades that will pause stress and help us manage it better. Here are some strategies:

* Understand that stress increases acidity in your body. Just ask the women in my hormone reset programs who quickly learn they cannot maintain a healthy alkaline state when they are stressed out or thinking negative thoughts. The most important solution here is to stick to a diet of mostly unprocessed foods with the right proportions of carbohydrates, protein, and healthy fats, and a wealth of alkalizing fresh vegetables and fruits. A diet that is made up of 80 percent alkaline and 20 percent acid foods makes for the healthiest diet. It is the key to supporting your hormones and staying healthy.

* Learn stress-management techniques such as deep breathing and practicing more positivity and appreciation (all help reduce stress!). Get a little extra sleep (so important!) for optimal health. Indulge in some vivid imagery of being in your favorite place in the world. Enjoy being in nature and go for a walk in the woods or on the beach when you can, or enjoy some quiet time with a sunrise or sunset.

Toxic Relationships

I could write a couple of books on this subject, but I'm going to keep it short. A toxic relationship could be a significant other who is emotionally or physically abusive, or both, a friend who puts you down more than they build you up, or a family member who constantly judges you. These people are hurting you and tearing down your self-esteem and confidence. They do not deserve a place in your life. Let them go, pause for a while, or put some distance between you and that person.

I love what author Bishop T. D. Jakes says about all this: "If someone can't treat you right, love you back, or see your worth, LET IT GO! If someone has angered you, LET IT GO! If you are involved in a wrong relationship or addiction, LET IT GO! If you are struggling with the healing of a broken relationship, LET IT GO!"

Start reflecting on relationships that tax you physically, mentally, and spiritually. Then . . . let them go.

A Negative Mindset

Your body and mind are interconnected, and you must take care of one in order to be able to take care of the other. In menopause, a positive mindset may not change "everything," but it will help your body produce happy hormones such as serotonin, dopamine, and endorphins. Collectively, this eases menopause discomforts and makes you feel better.

When you focus on the positives in your life and appreciate the goodness, you will reap many other health benefits, mainly in digestion, immunity, sleep, and mood, as well as so much more. Positivity can also help you be more resilient, so that when things in your life become challenging, you will be more able to cope.

To achieve a positive mindset, you must "mentally detox." Here's how:

Be grateful. Take 5 to 15 minutes and do some gratitude journaling every day. Ask yourself the questions, "What am I grateful for? What have I done to nourish my body and mind today? Where did I see love today?"

Indeed, much research over the past decade has found that people who consciously count their blessings tend to be happier and less depressed.

Take a moment to reflect. Do a bit of meditated reflection by asking yourself, "What could I have done better? How could I have been more loving?" This is so tremendously healing and upgrading to our quality of life.

As you reflect on what you are grateful for, you'll probably find that many of the things you write down in your journal are "external" to you. This is so awesome, as it means that your connections are what give you the most happiness. Connections are with the special people in your life, nature, your faith, pets, favorite activities, and so forth.

I am a creature of connection, so I always challenge myself at this time: "Was I focused on connection or disconnection during my day?" Try this yourself. Your answer to that might surprise you.

So often, as we get caught up in negative emotions and all the "things we desire"—and we forget all the wonderful relationships, moments, and things we have—we may even damage or lose our most precious connections.

Say "thank you" more often. I often mentally thank people. Think about someone who may have passed, but who was instrumental in your career choice or a favorite hobby. Or, mentally thank an early mentor or even that stranger who let you cut in line at the coffee shop one day! Picture the person and how he or she made you feel, and thank the person. It will make you feel great.

I also like to write thank you notes to people at this time, to let them know I appreciate them, whether that is because of something they did or simply because of who they are to me. And let me just say that there is something very gratifying about sitting down with paper and pen in hand, and actually writing a well-thought-out, from the heart, thank you note.

I encourage you to try this. Being thankful better realigns our priorities and helps us appreciate the people in our lives and the things they do.

Practice affirmations. Affirmations are statements that can reprogram your mind at the subconscious level and positively alter what you believe about yourself. They are also used to help us set intentions in order to create a future we desire—often in terms of attracting wealth, love, beauty, and happiness.

To help you get started, here are seven affirmations I use:

I am happy and joyful
I am content
I am energetic
I am productive
I am social and friendly
I am alert, my mind is focused
I feel good about my body

With a daily practice of affirmations, your mind and body start believing them. You will make better decisions. You will see a difference and become more happy, joyful, content, social, productive, friendly, and focused! Try it for a few weeks and you will see what I mean.

Tap into support. As you let go of what does not serve you, connect with those who support you—positive friends, family, and networks. One of the reasons I created The Girlfriend Doctor Club and my Keto-Green Community on Facebook is to give you that kind of positive support. A powerful "next right step" for you is to join these groups, where you will find inspiring success stories, amazing ideas for living the Keto-Green lifestyle, and an uplifting forum to air your thoughts about diet, hormone balance, and health in general. For information on how to join, see my Resources section.

Pausing Is Empowering

When you pause things in your life, you discover what works for you and what doesn't. You reclaim control over your own health destiny and this is supremely empowering. I encourage you to keep changing things up—from using the different nutritional plans in this book, to exercising in new ways, to even trying my special products such as Mighty Maca Plus or Julva. Whether it is through nutrition, hormonal balance, education, or all-natural products for women, I'm with you every step of the way to help you reboot your well-being and successfully continue your empowerment journey.

This is the end of the book, but really the beginning for you. Right now—today—is the perfect time to pause and re-engage your life. Real transformation comes as you move from behaviors and situations that don't support you to choices that do support you. Make that move.

YOU are worth the change. And remember, it is in the pauses of our lives where we find the magic!

Resources

RECOMMENDED TEST STRIPS AND OTHER TESTING TOOLS

Keto PH Test Strips: www.dranna.com

Hydrion pH Paper: www.amazon.com

KETO- MOJO Blood Ketone and Glucose Testing Meter Kit or PrecisionX-trablood ketone monitor: amazon.com

FreeStyle Libre 14- day system for continuing blood sugar monitoring (ask your doctor for a prescription)

SELF-TESTS AND OTHERS

dranna.com/evequiz

dranna.com/kegelvideo

dranna.com/oxytocinquiz

https://www.ultalabtests.com/drannacabeca
(for my recommended blood panels)

MENUPAUSE RECOMMENDED NUTRITIONAL SUPPLEMENTS

*Dr. Anna's Keto-Green® Alkaline Protein Shake

*Dr. Anna's Keto-Green® Shake

*Dr. Anna's Mighty Maca® Plus

*Dr. Anna's Omega Goodness

Vital- Zymes chewable digestive enzymes (www.klairelabs.com)

Complete Collagen Protein – Flavorless (www.drkellyann.com)

(*Available at www.dranna.com)

EXTRAS FOR WOMEN

Dr. Anna Cabeca's Julva feminine cream

Dr. Anna Cabeca's Balance cream

Join the Girlfriend Doctor Club (dranna.com)

Daily journal – download at dranna.com/menupause-extras

Check out other extras at: dranna.com/menupause-extras

RECOMMENDED KITCHENWARE AND COOKING TOOLS

Hamilton Beach Set 'n Forget Slow Cooker (It is free of lead, which many slow cookers contain.)

Nutribullet and Veggie Bullet

Radiant Life 14- Stage Biocompatible Water Purification System

Wusthof Knives

Vitamix

COOK BOOKS recommended by Dr. Anna

Overcoming Estrogen Dominance by Magdalena Wszelaki

The Low GI Slow Cooker by Mariza Snyder

The Mediterranean Method by Steven Masley, MD

Clean Southern Cuisine by Amanda Gipson

Sahtein by Middle East Cookbook

Lebanese Kitchen by Julie Taboulie

Zaitoun by Yasmin Khan

Acknowledgments

A cookbook like this takes time, creativity, and oh so much awareness, food testing and tasting, and inspiration—and all during an exciting time in my life. Since writing my second best-selling book, *Keto-Green 16*, I've moved from my family home in Saint Simons Island, Georgia, to Dallas, Texas. I lived in that home for 21 years with its large gourmet kitchen; now I have a lovely two-bedroom city condo with a small kitchen! Plus, I've spent many days and nights living in our horse trailer to attend weekend rodeos. Creating and experimenting with new recipes in these conditions has been challenging, to say the least!

I was assisted, thankfully, by my cousin Grace, a great cook and restaurateur. Like a sister to me, Grace visited me in Dallas and spent a month as a part of her own healing journey. She is an amazing and efficient cook who showed me how to work creatively in my small kitchen. I am forever grateful to Grace and her culinary creativity—and for being my initial test recipient with many of these meal plans.

I am also grateful to:

Karen Hall, who helped me get settled in Texas, organize the recipes, and assist me on the cookbook so that I used time efficiently, and so much more.

Maggie Greenwood-Robinson, who was instrumental in creating the framework for this cookbook. I can't say enough good things about her, and it would have been difficult to complete this masterpiece without her.

Nancy Hala, whose brand strategy was instrumental in bringing the Girlfriend Doctor brand to life.

My book team at Rodale, including my wonderful and supremely creative editor, Marnie Conchan, my visionary and super-talented agent Heather Jackson, and the rest of the dedicated staff there.

My friends and colleagues in my network who inspire me every day, including Angeli Akey, MD, Ellie Campbell, D.O., Magdalena Wzelaki, Cynthia Thurlow, N.P, J.J. Virgin, Steven Mastey, MD, Mindy Pelz, DC, and so many more.

My amazing daughters, Brittany, Amanda, Amira, and Ava, and my goddaughter Isabella. I am awed every moment by each one. They work with me and support my mission to help women around the world live their best lives. It has been beautiful to see them advocate for the next generation of women, helping them claim empowerment over their bodies in healthy, natural ways and sharing these messages, plans, the entire Keto-Green lifestyle, and my flagship product Julva and other products for women everywhere.

Immense, heartfelt gratitude goes to my team at the Girlfriend Doctor—I am truly blessed to have a wonderful, caring, and extremely professional work family who care about your health and personal empowerment as passionately as I do! Special gratitude goes out to Courtney Webster, Amy Stafford, Jamellette Diffoot, Lori Thomas, Jamy Gomes, Rossana Alvarado, Connie Calhoun, Yael Rosen, Edith Terolli, Lisa Curry, Josh Koerpel, Andreas Fried, Alom Mohammed, and Jason Ruona. They are friends and family to me. So much gratitude also goes to my team that is always ready to help, pitch in, and make things better, including Trent Walker, Sehrish Imran, Annie Epperley, Rachael Hanna, Shibani Subramanya, Yael Goodman, and Hannah Trygar, Kristen Matthews, and Jaime Bowen. I couldn't have created the gorgeousness and deliciousness of the recipes without Caroline Ely, who is truly a gifted chef and artist.

The Girlfriend Doctor Club members and Keto-Green community on Facebook to whom I am also very grateful for sharing their stories, recipes, challenges, and successes. Big hugs to the Unicorns out there in the world that inspire each other, especially my Unicorn Club girlfriends.

This cookbook is for all of you—and women and men around the world who want to break plateaus, reach new milestones, and obtain a healthier, better body today for a healthier tomorrow.

References

Chapter 1: Pause a Few Things on Your Menu to End Your Menopausal Symptoms

Christianson, M.S., et al. 2013. "Menopause Education: Needs Assessment of American Obstetrics and Gynecology Residents." *Menopause* 20: 1120–1125.

David, L.A., et. al. 2014. "Diet Rapidly and Reproducibly Gut Microbiome." *Nature* 505: 559–663. doi:10.1038/nature12820

Wolfe, J. 2018. "What Doctors Don't Know about Menopause." *AARP The Magazine*, August/September.

Chapter 2: How *MenuPause* Heals Your Body

Ghaemi-Hashemi, S.A., et al. 1998. "Benefits of the Middle Eastern Food Model on Women's Hormonal Balance." *Journal of the American Dietetic Association*, September, page A25.

Chapter 3: 6 Days to Menopausal Weight Loss, Energy, and Feeling Great

Brończyk-Puzoń, A., et al. 2015. "Guidelines for Dietary Management of Menopausal Women with Simple Obesity." *Przeglad Menopauzalny Menopause Review* 14: 48.

Compston, J. E., et al. 2011. "Obesity Is Not Protective against Fracture in Postmenopausal Women: GLOW." *American Journal of Medicine* 124: 1043–1050.

Dubnov-Raz, G., 2003. "Weight Control and the Management of Obesity after Menopause: The Role of Physical Activity." *Maturitas* 44: 89–101.

Dubnov-Raz, G., et al. 2007. "Diet and Lifestyle in Managing Postmenopausal Obesity." *Climacteric* 10: 38–41.

Lamerton, T. J., et al. 2018. "Overweight and Obesity as Major, Modifiable Risk Factors for Urinary Incontinence in Young to Mid-Aged Women: A Systematic Review and Meta-Analysis." *Obesity Reviews* 19: 1735–1745.

Lovejoy, J. C., et al. 2005. "Increased Visceral Fat and Decreased Energy Expenditure during the Menopausal Transition." *International Journal of Obesity* 32: 949.

Saccomani, S., et al. 2017. "Does Obesity Increase the Risk of Hot Flashes among Midlife Women?: A Population-Based Study." *Menopause* 24: 1065–1070.

Simkin-Silverman, L. R., et al. 2003. "Lifestyle Intervention Can Prevent Weight Gain during Menopause: Results from a 5-year Randomized Clinical Trial." *Annals of Behavioral Medicine* 26: 212–220.

Women's Health Network. "Menopause in Different Cultures." www.womenshealthnetwork.com/menopause-and-perimenopause/menopause-in-different-cultures.

Chapter 4: Keto-Green Extreme

Choi, Y., et al. 2013. "Indole-3-carbinol Directly Targets SIRT1 to Inhibit Adipocyte Differentiation." *International Journal of Obesity* 37: 881–884.

Fraser, G. E., et al. 2020. "Lower Rates of Cancer and All-Cause Mortality in an Adventist Cohort Compared with a US Census Population." *Cancer* 126: 1102–1111.

Horrobin, D. F. 1987. "Low Prevalences of Coronary Heart Disease (CHD), Psoriasis, Asthma and Rheumatoid Arthritis in Eskimos: Are They Caused by High Dietary Intake of Eicosapentaenoic Acid (EPA), a Genetic Variation of Essential Fatty Acid (EFA) Metabolism or a Combination of Both?" *Medical Hypotheses* 22: 421–428.

O'Keefe, J. H., and Harris, W. S. 2000. "From Inuit to Implementation: Omega-3 Fatty Acids Come of Age." *Mayo Clinic Proceedings* 75: 607–614.

Vohs, K. D., et al. 2013. "Rituals Enhance Consumption." *Psychological Science* 24: 1714–1721.

Chapter 5: Keto-Green Plant-Based Detox

Kiani, F., et al. 2006. "Dietary Risk Factors for Ovarian Cancer: the Adventist Health Study (United States)." *Cancer Causes Control* 17:137–146.

Nieman, D. C., et al. 1989. "Dietary Status of Seventh-Day Adventist Vegetarian and Non-Vegetarian Elderly Women." *Journal of the American Dietetic Association* 89 :1763–1769.

Orlich, M. J., et al. 2013. "Vegetarian Dietary Patterns and Mortality in Adventist Health Study 2." *JAMA Internal Medicine* 173: 1230–1238.

Rizzo, N. S., et al. 2013. "Nutrient Profiles of Vegetarian and Nonvegetarian Dietary Patterns."

Journal of the Academy of Nutrition and Dietetics 113: 1610–1619.

Schroeder, M. O. 2016. "What to Eat and Drink during Menopause." *U.S. News & World Report,* April 26.

Sisay, T., et al. 2020. "Changes in Biochemical Parameters by Gender and Time: Effect of Short-Term Vegan Diet Adherence." *PLoS One* 15: e0237065.

Tantamango, Y. M., et al. 2011. "Association between Dietary Fiber and Incident Cases of Colon Polyps: the Adventist Health Study." *Gastrointestinal Cancer Research* 4: 161–167.

Tonstad, S., et al. 2013. "Vegetarian Diets and Incidence of Diabetes in the Adventist Health Study-2." *Nutrition, Metabolism & Cardiovascular Diseases* 23: 292–299.

Chapter 6: The Carbohydrate Pause

Alali, W. Q., et al. 2010. "Prevalence and Distribution of Salmonella in Organic and Conventional Broiler Poultry Farms." *Foodborne Pathogens and Disease*, Epub July 9.

Ames, B. N. 2004. "Delaying the Mitochondrial Decay of Aging." *Annals of the New York Academy of Sciences* 1019: 406–411.

Choi, F. D., et al. 2019. "Oral Collagen Supplementation: A Systematic Review of Dermatological Applications." *Journal of Drugs in Dermatology* 18: 9–16.

Groenendijk, I., et al. 2019. "High Versus low Dietary Protein Intake and Bone Health in Older Adults: a Systematic Review and Meta-Analysis." *Computational and Structural Biotechnology Journal* 22: 1101–1112.

Gumbar, M. 2017. "A Sip above the Rest . . . Is Bone Broth All It's Boiled Up to Be?" *Product Update* 27: E39–E40.

Haentjens P. 2010. "Meta-Analysis: Excess Mortality after Hip Fracture among Older Women and Men." *Annals of Internal Medicine* 152: 380.

Halton, T. L., and Hu, F. B. 2004. "The Effects of High Protein Diets on Thermogenesis, Satiety and Weight Loss: A Critical Review." *Journal of the American College of Nutrition* 23: 373–385.

Kaplan, R. J., et al. 2001. "Dietary Protein, Carbohydrate, and Fat Enhance Memory Performance in the Healthy Elderly." *American Journal of Clinical Nutrition* 74: 687–693.

Layman, D. K., et al. 2006. "Potential Importance of Leucine in Treatment of Obesity and the Metabolic Syndrome." *Journal of Nutrition* 136: 319S–323S.

Le Floc'h, C., et al. 2015. "Effect of a Nutritional Supplement on Hair Loss in Women." *Journal of Cosmetic Dermatology* 14: 76–82.

Leidy, H. J., et al. 2015. "The Role of Protein in Weight Loss and Maintenance." *American Journal of Clinical Nutrition* 101: 1320S–1329S.

Liu, N., et al. 2019. "Stem Cell Competition Orchestrates Skin Homeostasis and Ageing." *Nature*, April 3.

McCuster, M., et al. 2010. "Healing Fats of the Skin: The Structural and Immunologic Roles of the Omega-6 and Omega-3 Fatty Acids." *Clinical Dermatology* 28: 440–451.

Skalny, A. V., et al. ??. "Zinc and Respiratory Tract infections: Perspectives for COVID19." (Review). *International Journal of Molecular Medicine* 46: 17–26.

Vellas, B. J., et al. 1997. "Changes in Nutritional Status and Patterns of Morbidity among Free-Living Elderly Persons: A 10-Year Longitudinal Study." *Nutrition* 13: 515–519.

Chapter 7: The Keto-Green Cleanse

Achamrah, N., et al. "Glutamine and the Regulation of Intestinal Permeability: from Bench to Bedside." *Current Opinion in Clinical Nutrition Metabolic Care* 20: 86–91.

Dietz, B. M., et al. 2016. "Botanicals and Their Bioactive Phytochemicals for Women's Health." *Pharmacological Reviews* 68: 1026–1073.

Faubion, S. S., et al. 2015. "Caffeine and Menopausal Symptoms: What Is the Association?" *Menopause* 22: 155–158.

Hegarty, V. M., et al. 2000. "Tea Drinking and Bone Mineral Density in Older Women." *American Journal of Clinical Nutrition* 71: 1003–1007.

Liu, Y., et al. 2017. "Therapeutic Potential of Amino Acids in Inflammatory Bowel Disease." *Nutrients* 9: 920.

Nair, A. R., et al. 2017. "Blueberry Supplementation Attenuates Oxidative Stress within Monocytes and Modulates Immune Cell Levels in Adults with Metabolic Syndrome: A Randomized, Double-Blind, Placebo-Controlled Trial." *Food & Function* 8: 4118–4128.

Newberg, A. B., et al. 2012. "A Pilot Study to Evaluate the Physiological Effects of a Spa Retreat That Uses Caloric Restriction and Colonic Hydrotherapy." *Integrative Medicine, A Clinician's Journal* 11: 26-32.

Rahimikian, F., et al. 2017. "Effect of Foeniculum vulgare Mill. (fennel) on Menopausal Symptoms in Postmenopausal Women: A Randomized, Triple-Blind, Placebo-Controlled Trial." *Menopause* 24: 1017–1021.

Rolls, B. J., et al. 2000. "Increasing the Volume of a Food by Incorporating Air Affects Satiety in Men." *American Journal of Clinical Nutrition* 72: 361–368.

Stefanopoulou, E., et al. 2014. "An International Menopause Society Study of Climate, Altitude, Temperature (IMS-CAT) and Vasomotor Symptoms in Urban Indian Regions." *Climacteric* 17: 417–424.

Wang, X., et al. 2020. "Tea Consumption and the Risk of Atherosclerotic Cardiovascular Disease and All-Cause Mortality: The China-PAR Project." *European Journal of Preventive Cardiology* 27: 1956–1963.

Whyte, A. R., et al. 2019. "Flavonoid-Rich Mixed Berries Maintain and Improve Cognitive Function Over a 6 h Period in Young Healthy Adults." *Nutrients* 6: 2685.

Chapter 8: The Carbohydrate Modification Plan

Donati, S., et al. 2009. "Menopause: Knowledge, Attitude and Practice among Italian Women." *Maturitas* 63: 246–252.

Sofer, S., et al. 2011. "Greater Weight Loss and Hormonal Changes after 6 Months Diet with Carbohydrates Eaten Mostly at Dinner." *Obesity* 19: 2006–2014.

Chapter 9: Keto-Green Extreme Recipes

Abshirini, M., et al. 2019. "Higher Intake of Dietary n-3 PUFA and Lower MUFA Are Associated with Fewer Menopausal Symptoms." *Climacteric* 22: 195–201.

Rahimikian, F., et al. 2017. "Effect of Foeniculum vulgare Mill. (fennel) on Menopausal Symptoms in Postmenopausal Women: A Randomized, Triple-Blind, Placebo-Controlled Trial." *Menopause* 24: 1017–1021.

Chapter 10: Keto-Green Plant-Based Detox Recipes

Rodriguez-Casado, A. 2016. "The Health Potential of Fruits and Vegetables Phytochemicals: Notable Examples." *Critical Reviews in Food Science and Nutrition* 56: 1097–1107.

Chapter 11: The Carbohydrate Pause Recipes

Fereidoon, S., and Priyatharini, A. 2018. "Omega-3 Polyunsaturated Fatty Acids and Their Health Benefits." *Annual Review of Food Science and Technology* 25: 345–381.

Fuller, N. R., et al. 2015. "Egg Consumption and Human Cardio-Metabolic Health in People with and without Diabetes." *Nutrients* 7: 7399–7420.

Roncero-Martin, R., et al. 2018. "Olive Oil Consumption and Bone Microarchitecture in Spanish Women." *Nutrients* 10: 968.

Wright, C. S., et al. 2018. "Effects of a High-Protein Diet Including Whole Eggs on Muscle Composition and Indices of Cardiometabolic Health and Systemic Inflammation in Older Adults with Overweight or Obesity: A Randomized Controlled Trial." *Nutrients* 10: 946.

Chapter 12: The Keto-Green Cleanse Recipes

Alasalvar, C., and Bolling, B. W. 2015. "Review of Nut Phytochemicals, Fat-Soluble Bioactives, Antioxidant Components and Health Effects." *British Journal of Nutrition* 113 Supplement 2: S68–S78.

White, D. 2021. "Healthy Uses for Garlic." *Nursing Clinics of North America* 56: 153–156.

Yadav, M., et al. 2010. "Medicinal and Biological Potential of Pumpkin: An Updated Review." *Nutrition Research Reviews* 23: 184–190.

Chapter 13: The Carbohydrate Modification Plan Recipes

Bower, A., et al. 2016. "The Health Benefits of Selected Culinary Herbs and Spices Found in the Traditional Mediterranean Diet." *Critical Reviews in Food Science and Nutrition* 56: 2728–2746.

Hewlings, S. J., and Kalman, D. S. 2017. "Curcumin: A Review of Its Effects on Human Health." *Foods* 6: 92.

Jakes, T.D. *Let It Go: Forgive So You Can Be Forgiven*, Atria Books, 2012.

Laribi, B., et al. 2015. "Coriander (Coriandrum sativum L.) and Its Bioactive Constituents." *Fitoterapia* 103: 9–26.

Parker, J., et al. 2018. "Therapeutic Perspectives on Chia Seed and Its Oil: A Review." *Planta Medica* 84: 606–612.

Index

Note: Page numbers in *italics* indicate photos or photo captions. Asterisks (*) following recipe titles indicate recipes shared from a different plan.

About the Author

Bestselling author, Anna Cabeca, DO, OBGYN, FACOG, is known nationally as The Girlfriend Doctor and is host of *The Girlfriend Doctor* show, where she welcomes experts and guests to the show to share their insights on how women can truly thrive in body, mind, and spirit. Dr. Anna is triple-board certified and a fellow of gynecology and obstetrics, integrative medicine, and anti-aging and regenerative medicine. She holds special certifications in functional medicine, sexual health, and bioidentical hormone replacement therapy. She lectures frequently on these topics throughout the world to large audiences.

Her first two highly acclaimed books, *The Hormone Fix* and *Keto-Green 16* are bestsellers. In addition, Dr. Anna is the creator of several popular virtual transformation programs—The Keto-Green Way to Breeze through Menopause, Sexual CPR, and Magic Menopause. She offers Keto-Green nutrition plans to online subscribers, is the founder of her Girlfriend Doctor Club, and the host of the vast Keto-Green community on Facebook.

A passionate health advocate for both women and men, Dr. Anna has appeared on numerous television shows and has been interviewed by ABC, CBS, and NBC. She also appeared in an episode of the *Real Housewives of Atlanta*. Sought after by various other media, Dr. Anna has been featured as a women's health, nutrition, weight loss, and hormone expert in *Shape Magazine*, *Woman's World*, *First for Women* magazine, *InStyle*, HuffPost, Mindbodygreen, and others.

Forbes Magazine reported on her success in creating and building a successful business around her flagship product Julva—an all-natural, over-the-counter cream that she developed to treat vaginal dryness and discomfort. Dr. Anna is also the creator of other top-selling health products such as Mighty Maca Plus.

Dr. Anna lives in Dallas, Texas, with her daughters, horses, and dogs.